The Nurse

In

Endocrinology

The Complete Guide

ALEXANDRE CAREWELL

Table of Contents

« *The delicate dance of hormones orchestrates the symphony of the body; endocrinology is the conductor.* »

Foreword :
THE IMPORTANCE OF ENDOCRINOLOGY AND ITS IMPACT ON OVERALL HEALTH.

Endocrinology, often described as the study of the body's chemical messengers, hormones, plays a vital role in understanding human health. In fact, this medical discipline goes beyond simple biological mechanisms to touch on almost every aspect of our physical, emotional and even mental well-being.

When you consider the complexity of our bodies, it quickly becomes apparent that even the slightest disturbance to one hormone can have a cascading effect, upsetting the delicate balance of our bodies. For example, thyroid hormones, produced in minuscule quantities, have a considerable influence on our metabolism, our energy and even our mood. Similarly, insulin, the pancreatic hormone, plays a central role in regulating our blood sugar levels, and any abnormality in its secretion or function can lead to diabetes, a disease with major systemic implications.

But beyond these physiological interactions, endocrinology also has a social and global impact. Take, for example, the current epidemic of diabetes and obesity. These pathologies, largely influenced by our modern lifestyles and environment, have become major public health concerns, involving not only medical issues, but also economic, social and ethical ones.

Endocrinology, in its quest to understand and treat hormonal imbalances, has the potential to improve the quality of life of billions of individuals. Whether through the management of growth disorders in children, thyroid dysfunction, the challenges of the menopause, or even more recent and sensitive issues such as the endocrine management of transgender people, this speciality embraces a diversity of subjects that reflects its centrality in the vast world of medicine.

Endocrinology is more than just the study of glands and their secretions. It represents a bridge between fundamental biology and clinical medicine, between the individual and his or her community, and between the present and the challenges of tomorrow. Recognising the importance of endocrinology means understanding that our well-being is intrinsically linked to this subtle hormonal balance which, like an invisible conductor, directs the complex symphony of our body.

Chapter 1:
INTRODUCTION TO ENDOCRINOLOGY

What is endocrinology?

Endocrinology is a specialised branch of medicine that studies the endocrine glands, the production and function of hormones, and the diseases and disorders associated with them. Hormones are essential chemical messengers that circulate in the bloodstream and regulate many of the body's vital functions, from growth and development to the way we use energy and the functioning of our reproductive organs.

Endocrine glands include the thyroid, parathyroid, pancreas, ovaries, testes, adrenal glands, pituitary gland and hypothalamus, to name but a few. Unlike exocrine glands, which release their secretions outside the body (such as the sweat or saliva glands), endocrine glands release their hormones directly into the bloodstream.

Endocrinology covers a wide range of conditions. The most common include diabetes (where insulin regulation is disrupted), thyroid disorders (such as hyperthyroidism or hypothyroidism), osteoporosis (affecting bone density), and hormonal imbalances related to reproduction or growth.

By its very nature, endocrinology is a highly integrative discipline, as hormones influence almost every organ and cell in the body. Endocrinologists, as specialists in this field, therefore play a key role in the diagnosis, treatment and management of hormonal disorders to ensure optimal function of the endocrine system and, by extension, the general well-being of the individual.

The endocrine glands and their roles.

Endocrine glands play a fundamental role in regulating various bodily functions. They secrete hormones directly into the bloodstream, which are then transported to various organs and tissues to exert their specific effects. Here is a list of the main endocrine glands and their associated functions:

- Pituitary gland :
    - Located at the base of the brain, it is often described as the "master gland" because it produces numerous hormones that regulate other endocrine glands.
    - Secretes growth hormone (GH), prolactin, thyrotropic hormones (TSH), corticotropins (ACTH), gonadotropins (LH and FSH) and vasopressin, among others.
- Hypothalamus :
    - Although it is part of the brain, it plays a crucial role in the endocrine system by regulating the pituitary gland through releasing or inhibiting hormones.
- Thyroid glands :
    - Located in the neck, they produce thyroid hormones (T3 and T4) which regulate metabolism, growth and development.
- Parathyroid   glands :
    - There are generally four of them, located behind the thyroid gland. They produce parathyroid hormone (PTH), which regulates calcium and phosphate in the blood.
- Adrenal glands :
    - Located above each kidney, they produce hormones such as cortisol, aldosterone and androgens. These hormones help regulate

metabolism, stress response, electrolyte balance and various sexual functions.

- Pancreas :
  - It is both an endocrine and an exocrine gland. Its endocrine function is performed by the islets of Langerhans, which produce insulin (regulates blood glucose levels) and glucagon (increases blood glucose levels).
- Ovaries (in women) :
  - They produce oestrogen, progesterone and small quantities of androgens. These hormones regulate the menstrual cycle, reproduction and certain secondary sexual characteristics.
- Testes (in men) :
  - They produce testosterone, which regulates spermatogenesis and male sexual characteristics.
- Pineal gland :
  - Located in the brain, it secretes melatonin, which regulates circadian rhythms and is involved in sleep cycles.

These glands and their respective hormones work closely together to maintain homeostasis in the body. The slightest imbalance can have significant repercussions on health, which underlines the importance of the endocrine system.

Common diseases and conditions.

The endocrine system, being essential for the regulation of many bodily functions, is subject to a variety of diseases and disorders. These disorders can result from excessive or insufficient production of hormones, or from a poor response of the target organs to these hormones. Here are some of the most common endocrine diseases and disorders:

- Diabetes :
    - **Type 1 diabetes**: The immune system attacks and destroys the β-cells of the islets of Langerhans in the pancreas, resulting in a lack of insulin production.
    - **Type 2 diabetes**: Insulin produced by the pancreas is not used properly by the body, leading to insulin resistance.
- Thyroid disorders :
    - **Hypothyroidism**: The thyroid gland does not produce enough thyroid hormone, leading to a slowdown in metabolism.
    - **Hyperthyroidism**: Overproduction of thyroid hormones, often due to Graves' disease.
    - **Goitre** : Abnormal increase in the size of the thyroid gland.
    - **Thyroid nodules**: Small growths or lesions in the thyroid gland.
    - Thyroid cancer.
- Parathyroid   gland disorders :
    - **Hyperparathyroidism:** excessive production of parathyroid hormone, often due to a tumour.
    - **Hypoparathyroidism**: Insufficient production of PTH.
- Adrenal gland disorders :
    - **Cushing's disease**: Excessive production of cortisol.
    - **Addison's disease**: Insufficient production of cortisol and aldosterone.
    - **Primary hyperaldosteronism:** too much aldosterone leading to a rise in blood pressure.
    - **Pheochromocytoma**: Rare tumour of the adrenal glands producing too much catecholamine.
- Pituitary disorders :
    - **Acromegaly**: Excessive production of growth hormone in adults.

- **Pituitary adenoma**: benign tumour of the pituitary gland.
  - **Hypopituitarism**: Insufficient production of one or more pituitary hormones.
- Reproductive disorders :
  - **Polycystic ovary syndrome (PCOS)**: Hormonal imbalance in women leading to ovarian problems.
  - **Hypogonadism**: Insufficient production of testosterone in men or oestrogen in women.
  - **Gynecomastia**: Abnormal development of breast tissue in men.
- Metabolic disorders :
  - **Osteoporosis**: loss of bone density, often linked to a reduction in oestrogen production in post-menopausal women.
- **Endocrine tumours**: Although rare, they can affect any endocrine gland.

Each of these diseases and conditions can have a variety of symptoms and requires a specific management approach. Early detection and appropriate intervention are essential to prevent complications and ensure optimal quality of life for patients.

The importance of the nurse's role in endocrinology.

The endocrinology nurse plays a pivotal role in the care of patients with endocrine disorders. Their role goes well beyond traditional nursing care, as endocrinology is a complex and multidimensional speciality. The importance of nursing in this context can be explored from a number of angles:

- **Patient education**: Endocrine diseases, such as diabetes or thyroid disorders, often require day-to-day management and a good understanding of the disease. Nurses are often at the forefront of educating patients about their condition, how to administer their medication, monitor their symptoms and recognise the warning signs of possible complications.

- **Treatment management**: Whether it's administering insulin for a diabetic patient or monitoring hormone levels for someone undergoing thyroid treatment, the nurse is essential in ensuring that medicines are given correctly and that patients are safe.

- **Liaison role**: The endocrinology nurse often acts as a link between the patient and the endocrinologist. He or she collects data, observes the evolution of symptoms and passes on this information, thus playing an essential role in the overall therapeutic strategy.

- **Psychological support**: Endocrine disease can have psychological repercussions. Diabetes, for example, can affect mood and quality of life. Nurses are often the health professionals closest to patients, offering support, listening and advice on managing the emotional aspects of endocrine disorders.

- **Continuous monitoring**: Advances in the field of endocrinology are constant. Nurses must keep up to date with the latest research, administration techniques and care recommendations to provide the best possible care.

- **Health promotion**: As part of prevention, particularly for diseases such as type 2 diabetes, nurses play a key role in raising awareness of the importance of a healthy lifestyle, promoting a balanced diet, regular physical activity and regular medical check-ups.

- **Endocrine emergencies**: Whether it's a thyrotoxic crisis or severe hypoglycaemia, the nurse is often the first responder, with the skills and training to stabilise the patient and prevent serious complications.

The endocrinology nurse is at the heart of patient care, combining technical skills, in-depth knowledge and a patient-centred approach. This unique combination makes them an indispensable part of the endocrinology care team.

Chapter 2:
DAILY REALITY
IN THE ENDOCRINOLOGY DEPARTMENT

Service structure and organisation.

The structure and organisation of an endocrinology department are designed to meet the specific needs of patients with endocrine disorders. The following is an outline of how such a service might be structured and organised:

- Specialist care units :
    - **Diabetes unit**: For the specific care of diabetic patients, with dedicated equipment such as insulin pumps, continuous glucose monitors, etc.
    - **Thyroid unit**: For patients with thyroid disorders.
    - **Adrenal gland and pituitary unit**: For rarer but equally important disorders.
    - **Bone metabolism unit**: For treating diseases such as osteoporosis.
    - **Reproduction unit**: Treatment of reproductive disorders linked to hormonal imbalances.
- Consultation rooms :
    - Where endocrinologists meet patients for follow-up consultations, initial examinations and ongoing assessments.
- Endocrinology laboratory :
    - Essential for hormone analyses and other related tests.

- Educational area :
    - A room dedicated to patient training, for example on diabetes management, self-administration of injections, etc.
- Integrated pharmacy :
    - To provide patients with all the specific medicines they need, such as hormones, insulin, etc.
- Administrative areas :
    - Offices for care coordination staff, case managers, etc.
- Research and development zone :
    - Some large endocrinology departments may have a research unit to study new therapies or treatment methods or to take part in clinical trials.
- Staff :
    - **Endocrinologists**: Doctors specialising in endocrinology.
    - **Specialist nurses**: Trained specifically in endocrinology.
    - **Dieticians**: Essential for managing diabetes and other disorders.
    - **Diabetes educators**: To train patients in diabetes management.
    - **Psychologists or counsellors**: To support patients in dealing with the emotional challenges of endocrine disorders.
    - **Medical assistants**: To help with consultations and procedures.
    - **Laboratory staff**: To carry out and analyse the tests.
- Technology and equipment :
    - At the cutting edge of monitoring, diagnosing and treating endocrine diseases.

- Care coordination :
- An efficient system for tracking appointments, treatments, care plans and communication between healthcare professionals.

The efficiency of an endocrinology department is based on a fluid organisation, where each element works in synergy to provide holistic patient care. Interdisciplinary collaboration is at the heart of this dynamic, ensuring that every aspect of the patient's health is taken into account.

Interaction with patients : initial contacts.

Interaction with patients, particularly during initial contacts, is an essential moment that shapes the therapeutic relationship and establishes a climate of trust. When a patient walks through the door of an endocrinology department for the first time, he or she is often filled with apprehension, questions and mixed feelings, ranging from hope to anxiety. It is at this precise moment that the importance of human contact is revealed in all its dimension.

As a healthcare professional, welcoming a patient means first and foremost recognising their uniqueness, their history and the issues surrounding their medical treatment. It means greeting them warmly, offering a reassuring smile, inviting them to express themselves freely while listening carefully to their words. This first meeting is a delicate dance in which clinical skill mingles with empathy, in which every question asked aims to understand not only the endocrine disorder in question, but also the emotional, social and psychological impact it has.

The discussion generally continues with a careful review of the patient's medical history, current symptoms and expectations, all wrapped up in clear, understandable language. At the same time, active listening plays a crucial role, as it allows us not only to detect what has not been said, but also to identify any concerns or fears that may be lurking in the background.

This first contact is also an opportunity to share information, to explain the next steps in the patient's care and to reassure him or her of the quality of the care that will be provided. It's a moment of exchange where each party gets to know the other, weaving the first threads of what promises to be a close and fruitful collaboration.

Initial contact with endocrinology patients is much more than a mere medical formality. They are the prelude to a therapeutic relationship based on trust, benevolence and mutual respect, the essential pillars for navigating together towards recovery.

Management of endocrine emergencies.

The management of endocrine emergencies is a crucial aspect of endocrine medicine, requiring rapid intervention, diagnostic precision and therapeutic expertise. These emergencies are situations where a hormonal imbalance or a complication of an endocrine disorder threatens the health or life of the patient and requires immediate treatment.

When a patient arrives at A&E with a clinical picture suggestive of an endocrine crisis, the first step is a rapid but thorough assessment of their condition. This often involves brief questioning to understand the recent history, including medication use, onset of symptoms and other possible triggers. At the same time, a vital assessment is carried out to check parameters such as blood pressure, heart rate, temperature and oxygen saturation.

Among the most common endocrine emergencies is the acute adrenal crisis, often linked to untreated adrenal insufficiency, manifested by severe weakness, hypotension and altered mental status. There is also the thyrotoxic crisis or thyroid storm, which is a severe exacerbation of hyperthyroidism. Hypoglycaemic coma, usually in diabetic patients, where a drastic fall in blood sugar levels can lead to loss of consciousness, is another frequent emergency. And of course we must not forget hyperosmolar coma and diabetic ketoacidosis, two serious complications of poorly controlled diabetes.

Once a diagnosis has been made or suspected, treatment must be initiated without delay. In most of these emergencies, time is of the essence, and every minute counts. Interventions can range from the simple administration of intravenous glucose for hypoglycaemia to more complex treatments, such as corticosteroids for an adrenal crisis or cooling therapy for a thyroid storm.

Following initial stabilisation of the patient, further investigation is carried out to determine the underlying cause of the emergency. This may include a range of laboratory tests, medical images and, sometimes, a consultation with a specialist endocrinologist.
The management of endocrine emergencies is a delicate balance between rapid action, clinical competence and holistic patient care. The ability to act effectively and make the right decisions in these stressful situations reflects not only the skill of the clinician, but also the depth and complexity of endocrinology as a medical specialty.

The specificities of night work.

Night work in the medical profession, and more widely in many fields, has unique characteristics that distinguish it from day work. Working when most of the world is asleep offers a different perspective, with its own challenges and rewards.

1. Disturbed circadian rhythm :
One of the greatest difficulties of working at night is the disruption of the circadian rhythm. Our biological clock is programmed to be awake during the day and asleep at night. Reversing this pattern can have consequences for our health, including increased fatigue, sleep disorders and an increased risk of certain diseases.

2. Increased requirements :
Although night-time may seem quieter in some establishments, there are often fewer staff, which means that each worker may have a heavier workload, be required to manage emergency situations with less support or carry out tasks outside their usual speciality.

3. Different working environment :
At night, the atmosphere is different. The corridors are quieter, the lights dimmer. This atmosphere can be both soothing and heavy. For some people, the calm of the night makes it easier to concentrate, while others may feel isolated or lonely.

4. Decision-making :
With fewer administrative and medical staff on site, night staff can often be faced with situations where quick, autonomous decisions are required, which can be both rewarding and stressful.

5. Interpersonal relations :
At night, the bonds between colleagues can become stronger. Faced with the unique challenges of night work, a camaraderie often develops between night workers. What's more, the often more intimate nature of night work can also allow for deeper and more meaningful interactions with patients.

6. Practical considerations :
Night workers often have to think about details that day workers don't consider. Where to find a meal in the middle of the night? How do you sleep during the day when the outside world is noisy and bright? How do you manage family and social obligations when you're working at cross-purposes?

7. Compensation and benefits :
In recognition of the challenges of night work, many employers offer night allowances or additional benefits for night staff.
Working at night is a very special experience, requiring adaptability and resilience. Although it's not for everyone, many find unexpected satisfaction and benefits in the calm and uniqueness of the night world.

Chapter 3:
TECHNIQUES AND PROCEDURES

Blood sampling and hormone tests.

Blood sampling and hormone testing are essential tools in the field of endocrinology, making it possible to assess and diagnose various conditions linked to hormonal imbalances. When the body displays symptoms suggestive of an endocrine disorder, it is often necessary to analyse the concentration of hormones in the blood to confirm or rule out a suspected diagnosis.

Blood samples :
The first stage of a hormone test is usually a blood sample. Taken by a nurse or laboratory technician, this involves inserting a needle into a vein, usually at the elbow, to collect a blood sample. The test is generally quick and, although sometimes uncomfortable, is usually well tolerated.

It should be noted that for some hormone tests, the time of sampling is crucial. For example, some hormones, such as cortisol, follow a circadian rhythm and may require sampling at a specific time of day. Other tests may require fasting or special conditions before sampling.

Hormone tests :
Once the blood sample has been collected, it is sent to the laboratory for analysis. Here are some of the most common hormone tests:

- Thyroid test :
    - TSH (thyroid stimulating hormone): To assess thyroid function.

- T3 and T4 (thyroid hormones): Measures the levels of hormones produced by the thyroid gland.
- Adrenal tests:
  - Cortisol: A hormone produced by the adrenal glands, particularly important in the response to stress.
  - Aldosterone and renin: Useful for assessing fluid balance and blood pressure.
- Reproduction tests :
  - LH and FSH: Gonadotropic hormones involved in reproduction.
  - Oestradiol, progesterone, testosterone: Female and male sex hormones.
- Pancreatic tests :
  - Insulin and C-peptide: To assess the function of pancreatic beta cells.
  - Glucose: To diagnose or monitor diabetes.
- Other tests :
  - Parathyroid hormone (PTH): Linked to the parathyroid glands and calcium metabolism.
  - Growth hormone: Important for growth and metabolism.

Once the tests have been completed, the results are interpreted by the endocrinologist, who assesses whether the hormone levels are within the normal range or whether they suggest an imbalance or condition. This information is essential for making a precise diagnosis and guiding the patient's treatment.

Treatment administration.

The administration of treatments in endocrinology is a delicate task, requiring a thorough understanding of endocrine disorders and the drugs used to treat them. Hormones, by their very nature, play a regulatory role in the body, and their replacement or modulation must be carried out with precision to avoid potentially damaging imbalances.

1. Methods of administration :
   - **Orally**: Many endocrine treatments are administered orally in the form of tablets or capsules, such as thyroid hormones or certain diabetes medications.
   - **Injection**: Some treatments, such as insulin or growth hormone, are administered by injection, either subcutaneously, intramuscularly or, more rarely, intravenously.
   - **Infusion pumps**: For example, insulin pumps that continuously administer insulin at a basal rate and deliver extra doses at mealtimes.
   - **Implants and sustained-release devices**: Such as testosterone implants or intrauterine devices that release progestins.
   - **Topically**: in the form of gels or patches, like certain testosterone- or oestrogen-based treatments.

2. Dosage :
Accurate dosing is essential. An overdose or underdose can have serious consequences. Regular monitoring of blood levels of a hormone or drug may be necessary to adjust the dosage.

3. Monitoring and adaptation :
The efficacy and tolerability of the treatment must be monitored regularly. This may involve blood tests, physical examinations and discussions with the patient to identify any side effects or persistent symptoms.

4. Patient education :
It is crucial to educate the patient on the importance of taking the treatment as prescribed, recognising the signs of

overdose or underdose, and knowing when to seek advice. For some treatments, such as insulin, the patient may also need training in injection technique.

5. Drug interactions :
Hormones can interact with other drugs that the patient may be taking. It is therefore essential to monitor these interactions and adjust treatments accordingly.

6. Psychological aspects :
Taking hormones can affect mood and behaviour. It is important to monitor and support the patient in these areas, in collaboration with other healthcare professionals if necessary.

The administration of endocrinology treatments is a complex task requiring constant attention, medical expertise and close collaboration with the patient. Every patient is unique, and treatment must be personalised accordingly to ensure the best possible results.

Preventing complications.

Preventing complications is an essential aspect of the management of endocrine disorders. Given the regulatory nature of hormones on many bodily functions, imbalances or inappropriate treatments can lead to a series of complications, some of them serious. It is therefore essential to adopt preventive strategies.

1. Patient education and training :
One of the first steps in preventing complications is to ensure that patients are well informed about their disease, the treatments prescribed and the behaviour they should adopt. For example, a diabetic patient needs to be trained in self-monitoring of blood sugar, how to adjust the insulin

dose, how to recognise the signs of hyperglycaemia or hypoglycaemia, and how to intervene.

2. Regular medical check-ups :
Close monitoring allows potential disturbances to be identified and treated quickly. This may include regular consultations with an endocrinologist, periodic blood tests and other diagnostic examinations.

3. Therapeutic adherence :
It is essential that patients follow the prescribed treatment plan, whether this involves taking medication, adopting lifestyle modifications or following other medical recommendations. Non-adherence can significantly increase the risk of complications.

4. Healthy lifestyles :
Many endocrine disorders, such as type 2 diabetes or osteoporosis, can be influenced by lifestyle. Encouraging a balanced diet, regular physical activity and limiting alcohol consumption and smoking can help prevent complications.

5. Care coordination :
Collaboration between different health professionals, such as GPs, endocrinologists, dieticians, specialist nurses and psychologists, among others, can ensure holistic patient care.

6. Identifying and managing risk factors :
This may include blood pressure control, weight management, lipid profile monitoring, and other measures to reduce the risks associated with certain endocrine disorders.

7. Vaccinations and infection prevention :
For example, diabetic patients are more susceptible to infections. Regular vaccinations, such as the flu vaccine or

pneumococcal vaccination, may therefore be recommended.

<u>8. Raising awareness of the importance of monitoring :</u>
Motivate patients to take an active part in their care, to recognise the importance of follow-up visits and not to overlook unusual symptoms.

Preventing complications in endocrinology is a proactive approach that involves both healthcare professionals and patients. It is based on sound education, regular monitoring, therapeutic adherence and comprehensive management, with the aim of guaranteeing optimal quality of life for the patient while minimising the risks associated with the disease and treatment.

Therapeutic patient education.

Therapeutic patient education is a collaborative journey between healthcare professional and patient, focused on empowerment and actively taking charge of their health. It goes far beyond the simple transmission of information; it aims to equip patients with the skills and knowledge they need to manage their disease, improve their quality of life and prevent complications.

At the heart of this educational approach is the recognition that the individual is not simply the recipient of instructions, but a full player in his or her own care. It is in this context that a rich, two-way dialogue is established, in which patients are encouraged to ask questions, share their concerns, and express their needs and aspirations relating to their condition.

Therapeutic education is not limited to understanding the disease or the treatment prescribed. It also encompasses the ability to recognise and act on symptoms, to understand the importance of adherence to treatment, to manage the psychological and emotional aspects of the disease, and to adopt healthy lifestyles. Each educational session is therefore an opportunity for the patient to acquire or reinforce these skills, with the support and expertise of the healthcare team.

The role of the healthcare professional in this process is crucial. As well as providing accurate, up-to-date information, they must also be good listeners, show empathy, adapt their discourse to the patient's level of understanding and encourage the patient's active participation. It's a respectful exchange in which the patient feels valued and supported.
As patients immerse themselves in this educational process, the benefits become clear. Greater autonomy in managing the disease, fewer hospitalisations and complications, improved quality of life and greater satisfaction with the care received are just some of the many benefits.

Therapeutic patient education is a harmonious dance, in which clinical expertise blends with humanity, and in which every step, every movement, is directed towards an ultimate goal: the well-being and fulfilment of the patient in the face of his or her condition.

Chapter 4:
DISEASES AND TREATMENT

Diabetes mellitus : a global epidemic.

• Understanding the disease.

Diabetes mellitus is a condition that is attracting a great deal of attention, and with good reason: it is a chronic disease that is on the rise worldwide, affecting millions of people of all ages and from all walks of life. Understanding this disease means first and foremost delving into the inner workings of our bodies, to discover the mechanisms that regulate the level of sugar in our blood.

At the heart of our body, the pancreas plays a key role. This gland, nestled behind the stomach, produces an essential hormone: insulin. Like an orchestra conductor, insulin sets the tempo and regulates the amount of glucose, or sugar, in the blood. After eating, when our food is converted into glucose, it is insulin that comes into play to enable the cells in our body to use this glucose as a source of energy or to store it for later use.

Diabetes mellitus occurs when this delicate process is disrupted. There are two main types:

- **Type 1 diabetes**: Here, the body produces little or no insulin because the cells in the pancreas that produce it are destroyed by the patient's immune system. This form of diabetes generally appears in young people, hence its former name of "juvenile diabetes". The exact reasons for this autoimmune destruction are still being studied, but genetic and environmental factors appear to be involved.

- **Type 2 diabetes**: Much more common, this type of diabetes is characterised by insulin resistance. This means that, although the pancreas produces insulin, the body does not respond effectively to it. Over time, the pancreas may no longer produce enough insulin to maintain normal blood sugar levels. This form of diabetes is often associated with age, obesity, a sedentary lifestyle and genetic factors.

The consequences of uncontrolled blood sugar levels are numerous and can affect almost every organ. Long-term complications include heart, kidney, eye and nerve problems, among others. In addition, wounds can take longer to heal, and the risk of infection is increased.
Common symptoms of diabetes, whether type 1 or type 2, include intense thirst, frequent urination, persistent fatigue, unexplained weight loss (more common in type 1), blurred vision and excessive hunger.

The management of diabetes is based on a combination of medication (such as insulin or oral antidiabetics), a balanced diet, regular physical activity and careful monitoring of blood sugar levels.
In short, diabetes mellitus is a major medical and social challenge. Understanding and managing it requires a comprehensive, multidisciplinary approach, putting the patient at the centre of our concerns, while drawing on scientific and medical advances to offer increasingly personalised and effective care.

• Care and intervention.

Diabetes mellitus care and interventions are an essential part of the management of this complex disease. The key lies in a comprehensive, individualised approach for each patient, ensuring optimal glycaemic control while preserving quality of life.

1. Monitoring blood glucose levels :
This is the central element of diabetes monitoring. Regular measurement of blood sugar levels, whether by home

monitoring devices, continuous sensors or laboratory tests such as HbA1c (which gives an average glucose level over 3 months), enables treatment to be adjusted and complications to be prevented.

2. Anti-diabetic drugs :
  - **Insulin therapy**: For patients with type 1 diabetes and some patients with type 2 diabetes, the administration of insulin is essential. It can be administered by conventional injections or insulin pumps.
  - **Oral antidiabetics**: Used mainly for type 2 diabetes, they act in various ways, such as increasing insulin secretion, improving insulin sensitivity or slowing down the absorption of glucose by the intestine.

3. Dietary advice :
A balanced, appropriate diet is fundamental to managing diabetes. The emphasis is on a diet rich in fibre and low in simple sugars, with a controlled intake of complex carbohydrates. A specialist dietician can provide invaluable advice on food choices, portion sizes and taking into account the impact of meals on blood sugar levels.

4. Physical activity :
Regular exercise helps to improve insulin sensitivity, control blood sugar levels and maintain a healthy weight. Recommendations are tailored to each patient's abilities and preferences.

5. Prevention and management of complications :
This includes regular consultations with specialists such as ophthalmologists to monitor diabetic retinopathy, podiatrists for foot care, or nephrologists to monitor kidney function.

6. Therapeutic education :
Teach patients how to manage their disease, adjust their treatment, recognise and treat hypo- or hyperglycaemic

episodes, and adopt behaviours that are beneficial to their health.

7. Psychological support :
When faced with a chronic diagnosis, it is essential to address the emotional aspect. Psychological support, either individually or in a group, can help manage the stress, anxiety and depression associated with the illness.

8. Technological innovations :
Nowadays, there are tools such as continuous glucose monitors, mobile tracking applications and smart insulin pumps that can greatly improve diabetes management.

Each intervention or treatment is tailored to the patient's individuality, type of diabetes, needs and lifestyle. Close collaboration between the patient, the endocrinologist and the entire medical team is the cornerstone of successful management of diabetes mellitus, with the aim of achieving optimal glycaemic control and a full and fulfilling life.

• **Management of hypoglycaemia and hyperglycaemia.**

Managing hypoglycaemia and hyperglycaemia is crucial for people with diabetes. These fluctuations in blood sugar levels can have consequences ranging from mild discomfort to potentially fatal if they are not treated quickly and effectively.

Hypoglycaemia :
Hypoglycaemia occurs when blood glucose levels are abnormally low, generally below 70 mg/dL, although this threshold can vary from person to person.
- **Common symptoms:** Trembling, sweating, dizziness, hunger, irritability, palpitations, confusion, weakness,

slurred speech, drowsiness, and in severe cases, loss of consciousness or convulsions.

- Management :
- The "15" rule is often taught: eat 15 grams of fast-acting carbohydrate (for example, 3-4 lumps of sugar, a glass of orange juice or glucose jelly) and then check your blood sugar after 15 minutes. If it remains low, eat 15g of carbohydrate again.
- Avoid eating high-fat foods to correct hypoglycaemia, as they slow down the absorption of glucose.
- Once blood sugar levels have stabilised, if the next meal is more than an hour away, eat a balanced snack to avoid another hypoglycaemia.

Hyperglycaemia :

Hyperglycaemia refers to abnormally high blood glucose levels. Although there may be individual variations, it is generally considered to be present when blood glucose levels exceed 180 mg/dL after a meal.

- **Common symptoms**: Excessive thirst, frequent urination, fatigue, blurred vision, slow wound healing, and in severe cases, rapid breathing, fruity breath odour, and loss of consciousness.
  - Management :
  - Check blood sugar levels regularly and adjust treatment according to your doctor's recommendations.
  - Drink plenty of water to help eliminate excess glucose through the urine.
  - Avoid sugary drinks or foods that could raise blood sugar levels even higher.
  - Consult a doctor if blood sugar levels remain high or if symptoms of ketosis develop (fruity smell on the breath, nausea, vomiting, abdominal pain).

For both situations, it is essential to be well informed and prepared. This means always having glucose or a source of carbohydrates available to treat hypoglycaemia, or having the means to check blood sugar levels if symptoms of hyperglycaemia occur. In addition, regular communication with healthcare professionals and ongoing diabetes education can help prevent and effectively manage these blood sugar episodes.

Thyroid disorders.

• Hyperthyroidism and hypothyroidism.

Hyperthyroidism and hypothyroidism are two common disorders of the endocrine system that affect the function of the thyroid gland, a butterfly-shaped organ located at the base of the neck. This gland produces thyroid hormones, mainly thyroxine (T4) and triiodothyronine (T3), which play a key role in regulating the body's energy metabolism.

Hyperthyroidism :
Hyperthyroidism refers to an overproduction of thyroid hormones.
- Common causes:
    - Graves' disease: an autoimmune disease in which the body produces antibodies that over-stimulate the thyroid gland.
    - Toxic multinodular goitre: presence of nodules or non-cancerous tumours which produce too much thyroid hormone.
    - Thyroiditis: an inflammation of the thyroid gland, which sometimes releases too many stored hormones.
- Common symptoms:
    - Palpitations, tremors, irritability.

- Unexplained weight loss, increased appetite.
- Excessive sweating, heat intolerance.
- Diarrhoea or frequent Feces.
- Exorbated eyes or eye irritation (particularly in Graves' disease).
- Fatigue.
- Management and processing :
    - Antithyroid drugs (e.g. methimazole).
    - Radioactive iodine to reduce the size and activity of the gland.
    - Surgery (thyroidectomy) in certain cases.
    - Beta-blockers to reduce certain symptoms.

Hypothyroidism :
It describes a situation where the thyroid gland does not produce enough hormones.
- Common causes:
    - Hashimoto's thyroiditis: an autoimmune disease in which the thyroid gland is progressively destroyed.
    - Treatment for hyperthyroidism (radioactive iodine or surgery) which excessively reduces thyroid activity.
    - Certain drugs, such as lithium.
    - Lack of iodine in the diet.
- Common symptoms:
    - Fatigue, weakness.
    - Unexplained weight gain, difficulty losing weight.
    - Dry skin, brittle hair and hair loss.
    - Feeling of cold.
    - Constipation.
    - Low mood or depression.
- Management and processing :
    - Levothyroxine: a drug that replaces the missing thyroid hormone.

- Regular monitoring of thyroid hormone levels to adjust the dose of levothyroxine if necessary.
- Dietary considerations to ensure adequate iodine intake.

Understanding these two disorders requires an integrated approach, taking into account not only the clinical symptoms, but also the emotional and psychological needs of the patient. Adherence to treatment, regular monitoring and patient education are essential for optimal management of both hyperthyroidism and hypothyroidism.

• Thyroid cancer.

Thyroid cancer, although less common than other types of cancer, has seen an increase in prevalence in recent years, often attributed to improved detection techniques. The thyroid, a butterfly-shaped endocrine gland located at the base of the neck, plays a crucial role in regulating the body's metabolism through the production of hormones.

Types of thyroid cancer :
- **Papillary carcinoma**: This is the most common type. It is generally slow-growing and develops in the follicular cells.
- **Follicular carcinoma**: Less common than papillary carcinoma, it also develops in follicular cells and can spread further throughout the body.
- **Medullary carcinoma**: This starts in the C (parafollicular) cells of the thyroid, which produce the hormone calcitonin. Its progression is generally more aggressive than that of papillary or follicular carcinomas.
- **Anaplastic carcinoma: This is** a rare but very aggressive type of thyroid cancer that progresses rapidly.

<u>Symptoms</u> :
Many thyroid cancers initially cause no symptoms. However, as they progress, signs may appear:
- A mass or nodule in the neck, often detected during a physical examination or by chance during imaging.
- Pain in the throat or neck.
- Changes in voice, in particular a hoarse voice.
- Difficulty swallowing.
- Shortness of breath or wheezing.
- Swelling of the lymph nodes in the neck.

<u>Diagnosis</u> :
- **Thyroid ultrasound**: This is the first step in assessing the size and structure of the nodules.
- **Fine needle biopsy**: Used to analyse samples of thyroid tissue to detect the presence of cancerous cells.
- **Blood tests**: To assess thyroid function and measure thyroid hormone levels.
- **Thyroid scan**: Used to determine the "hot" or "cold" nature of a nodule, which can help determine whether it is likely to be benign or malignant.

<u>Treatment</u> :
Treatment depends on the type and stage of the cancer, as well as the patient's general health:
- **Surgery**: Total or partial thyroidectomy is commonly performed to remove all or part of the thyroid gland.
- **Radioactive iodine therapy (RAI):** Used after surgery to destroy any remaining thyroid cells.
- **Hormonal therapy**: To replace thyroid hormones and inhibit the secretion of TSH, which could stimulate the growth of cancer cells.
- **Radiotherapy or chemotherapy**: Generally reserved for more aggressive or advanced cancers.

<u>Forecast</u> :
The prognosis for thyroid cancer is generally favourable, particularly for young individuals and for cancers detected at an early stage. Papillary and follicular carcinomas are

often curable, while medullary and anaplastic carcinomas present greater challenges.

Prevention, early detection and appropriate management are essential to ensure the best possible outcome for people with thyroid cancer. Research also continues to make advances in understanding and treating this disease.

• Post-operative follow-up.

Post-operative follow-up is a crucial step after any surgical procedure, including thyroid surgery. It aims to monitor the patient's recovery, detect and manage any complications, and ensure that treatment goals are met, particularly in the context of thyroid cancer surgery.

1. Immediate surveillance :
   - **Pain**: Pain and discomfort at the incision site are common and can be managed with prescribed analgesics.
   - **Vocal function**: Thyroid surgery can sometimes affect the laryngeal nerves, so it is important to monitor any change in voice or difficulty in speaking.
   - **Calcium**: Calcium levels may fall if the parathyroid glands adjacent to the thyroid are damaged during surgery, causing numbness, tingling or muscle cramps.

2. Medium and long-term monitoring :
   - **Healing**: The surgeon will assess the scar, making sure it is healing properly and possibly suggesting treatments or recommendations to minimise its appearance.
   - **Thyroid function**: After a total thyroidectomy, patients will probably need to take thyroid replacement medication for life. Regular blood tests will enable the dose to be adjusted.
   - **Cancer monitoring**: For those who have undergone surgery for thyroid cancer, monitoring is essential to detect any recurrence. This may include blood tests

to measure thyroglobulin levels, ultrasound scans and sometimes thyroid scans.

- **Radioactive iodine therapy**: Some patients may require post-operative radioactive iodine treatment to eliminate residual thyroid cells or to treat recurrent cancer.

3. Complications and management :

- **Hypocalcaemia**: If the parathyroid glands have been affected, calcium and vitamin D supplements may be necessary.
- **Vocal complications**: Vocal therapies may be offered if the patient has persistent problems with their voice.
- **Lymphedema**: A build-up of lymph fluid can sometimes occur in the neck, requiring physiotherapy or other interventions.

4. Emotional and psychological support :

Cancer surgery and diagnosis can be emotionally distressing. Psychological care, through therapy sessions, support groups or consultations with specialists, can be beneficial.

5. Patient education and empowerment :

Provide detailed information on post-operative management, recognising the signs of complications, the importance of taking medication regularly, and dietary recommendations.

Post-operative monitoring is a collaboration between the patient and the medical team, focused on recovery, preventing complications and ensuring the best possible quality of life. Every step, from immediate monitoring to regular long-term check-ups, is essential to ensure the best possible outcome for the patient.

Conditions affecting the adrenal, pituitary and parathyroid glands.

The endocrine glands play a fundamental role in regulating bodily functions through the production of hormones. Among these, the adrenal glands, pituitary gland and parathyroid glands are essential for physiological balance. Conditions affecting these glands can lead to a series of metabolic disorders.

Adrenal glands :

Located above each kidney, they produce a number of hormones, including cortisol, aldosterone and androgens.

- **Hypercorticism:** Commonly known as Cushing's syndrome, it is characterised by an overproduction of cortisol. Symptoms: obesity centred on the trunk, rounded face, purple stretch marks, muscle and bone weakness, high blood pressure.
- **Hypofunction (or adrenal insufficiency):** Known as Addison's disease, it results from insufficient production of cortisol and often aldosterone. Symptoms: fatigue, weight loss, dark patches on the skin, low blood pressure.

Pituitary gland :

Located at the base of the brain, this small gland is often called the "master gland" because it regulates many other endocrine glands.

- **Pituitary adenoma:** A benign tumour that can press on neighbouring tissues or produce an excess of hormones. Symptoms depend on the excess hormone.
- **Pituitary insufficiency:** Reduced production of one or more pituitary hormones. Symptoms depend on which hormone is insufficient.

<u>Parathyroid</u> :

Four small glands located behind the thyroid gland, they regulate calcium and phosphate in the body.

- **Hyperparathyroidism**: results in an overproduction of parathyroid hormone, which increases calcium levels. Symptoms: bone weakness, kidney stones, abdominal pain and fatigue.
- **Hypoparathyroidism**: Insufficient production of parathyroid hormone, leading to low levels of calcium in the blood. Symptoms: muscle cramps, tingling, muscle spasms, dry hair, brittle nails.

Management of these conditions depends on the underlying cause and associated symptoms. It may include drugs to replace or inhibit hormone production, surgery to remove tumours or glands, and targeted therapies to treat specific symptoms.

The complexity of these conditions highlights the importance of a multidisciplinary approach to treatment, involving endocrinologists, surgeons, radiologists and other specialists to ensure the best possible outcome for each patient. Regular monitoring is also essential, as hormonal balance is delicate and patients' needs can change over time.

Chapter 5:
COMMUNICATION AND OLLABORATION

Communicating effectively
with patients and their families.

Communicating with patients and their families is a delicate art that is deeply intertwined with the science of medicine. In the hustle and bustle of hospitals, clinics and doctors' surgeries, where technology, diagnosis and treatment are at the forefront, it's crucial not to neglect the human side of healing. The words we choose, the tone we use and even our body language can have a significant impact on how patients perceive their condition, adhere to their treatment and, ultimately, heal.

Establishing a relationship of trust is the first step. This starts with active listening, giving full and undivided attention to what the patient or their family is saying. It's about deciphering not just the words, but also the underlying emotions: fear, uncertainty, hope. By validating these feelings, we humanise the medical experience and recognise that behind every patient lies a story, dreams, fears and aspirations.

It is also essential to provide information that is clear and understandable. Medical terms can sometimes seem like a foreign language to the uninitiated. Simplifying jargon, using analogies or metaphors and ensuring that the patient and their family have a clear understanding of the condition, the treatment plan and any side effects or complications is vital.
But communicating doesn't just mean talking; it also means asking questions and encouraging patients and their families to ask their own. By creating an open

dialogue, concerns can be expressed and uncertainties clarified.

Communication is also about what is left unsaid. Sometimes a reassuring touch, a moment's silence or a simple gesture of empathy can convey more than words. It's also essential to be aware of cultural differences, beliefs and values that can influence perceptions of illness and treatment.

Finally, collaboration is key. Every patient is unique, as are their families. By working together as a team, doctors, nurses, patients and families can ensure that the care provided is not only technically appropriate, but also deeply humane.

Communicating effectively with patients and their families is not a luxury, but a necessity. It is the heart of medicine, and perhaps the most powerful healing tool at our disposal.

Managing complex cases: coordination with other departments.

In the medical world, where each speciality deals with distinct facets of health, the management of complex cases often requires close coordination between different services. This interdisciplinary collaboration is crucial to providing holistic care, ensuring a smooth transition of care, avoiding duplication and optimising the use of resources.

Complex cases are generally defined by a combination of multiple health problems, which may be both chronic and acute, physical and psychological. For example, a patient with diabetes, hypertension or depression who has just undergone surgery requires the expertise of several specialists: an endocrinologist, a cardiologist, a psychiatrist, a surgeon and probably other health professionals.

At the heart of case management is the pivotal role of the GP or coordinating nurse. They often play the role of "orchestra conductor", drawing up the care plan, ensuring that all the necessary interventions are scheduled and followed up, and ensuring communication between all the specialists involved.

But that's not all. In addition to specialist consultations, coordination often also involves rehabilitation or physiotherapy services, dieticians, social workers, psychologists, and sometimes more specialised services such as oncology, nephrology or cardiology. When a patient is admitted to hospital, this coordination extends to the ward team, including nurses, Caregivers, pharmacists and other health professionals.

Communication is therefore the cornerstone of this coordination. It must be clear, precise and patient-centred. Electronic medical records, multidisciplinary meetings and structured referral systems are essential tools for facilitating this communication.

However, as important as these tools are, they are no substitute for the human element. The ability to listen, to understand the perspectives of other specialists, and above all, to put the patient at the centre of all decisions, is what differentiates simple coordination from effective coordination.

Managing complex cases through inter-departmental coordination is a challenge that requires both technical expertise and interpersonal skills. It's a delicate ballet, where each player needs to know their role and be ready to adapt according to the patient's needs. But when it's done properly, the results can be transformative, offering patients comprehensive care that addresses all their concerns and needs.

Chapter 6:
PAEDIATRIC ENDOCRINOLOGY

Specific challenges
children and teenagers.

Caring for children and teenagers presents unique challenges that go far beyond those encountered with adults. Not only are their bodies and minds constantly changing, but they also have to navigate the tumult of life transitions, while trying to understand their own identity and place in the world.

1. Growth and development: Unlike adults, children are constantly growing and developing. This means that their medical, nutritional and emotional needs can change rapidly. Medicines and treatments often need to be adjusted according to their size and age, and what works at one time may not be appropriate a few months later.

2. Communication: Children and teenagers do not always have the skills or vocabulary to express their feelings, pains or concerns. So we often have to read between the lines, use age-appropriate communication techniques, and sometimes rely more on observation than words.

3. Consent and autonomy: Striking the right balance between respecting a teenager's autonomy and the need for parental consent can be complex, especially when it comes to sensitive issues such as sexual health, mental health or gender transition care.

4. Issues specific to adolescence: Adolescents face a myriad of unique challenges, such as peer pressure, body image concerns, substance experimentation, identity conflicts and academic challenges. These issues can influence and be influenced by their overall health.

5. Family impact: The illness or disorder of a child or adolescent often has an impact on the whole family. Parents may feel guilty, frustrated or overwhelmed. Siblings may feel jealous or neglected. Family support is therefore crucial, as is taking family dynamics into account in the care plan.

6. Continuity of care: As children grow older, they often need to move from specialist paediatric services to adult services. This transition can be confusing and stressful for young patients who have built up trusting relationships with their paediatric providers.

7. Socio-economic and educational issues: Children's and young people's health problems can affect their schooling, social relationships and extra-curricular activities. It is crucial to integrate a holistic approach to ensure that they are not only "healthy", but that they can also thrive in their everyday environment.

To meet these challenges, it is imperative to adopt a child- and family-centred approach, where care is tailored to the unique needs of each patient, taking into account both their stage of development and their socio-cultural context. This requires specialist training, a great deal of empathy and the ability to work closely with a multidisciplinary team.

Transition from paediatric to adult endocrinology.

The transition from paediatric to adult endocrinology is a critical stage for many young patients with endocrine disorders. This transition is not just about moving from one doctor or environment to another, but involves a profound change in the way patients are involved in their care, and in the expectations and responsibilities placed on them.

1. Preparing for the transition :
Preparing for this transition must start well before the patient leaves the paediatric ward. This means educating the young person about their illness, making sure they understand the importance of their treatment, and familiarising them with the differences between paediatric and adult care.

2. Increased responsibility :
In paediatric care, parents or guardians play a central role in the patient's care. However, in the adult system, patients are expected to take on more responsibility, managing appointments, medication and follow-up.

3. Differences in approach to care :
Paediatric endocrinology often focuses on issues related to growth, development and puberty. Adult endocrinology, on the other hand, addresses concerns that can be more complex, relating to reproduction, advanced age, the long-term complications of endocrine disorders and the associated diseases that develop with age.

4. Psychosocial needs :
Young adults may have specific concerns related to their illness, such as the impact on their relationships, sexuality, career and desire to start a family. These concerns require appropriate care and support.

5. Ongoing support :
The transition should not be an abrupt 'jump' from one service to another, but rather a fluid process with ongoing support. This could include joint consultations with paediatricians and adult specialists or education sessions to familiarise the patient with the new care setting.

6. Care coordination :
Effective communication between paediatric and adult teams is crucial. Medical records, treatment histories and other relevant information must be passed on seamlessly to ensure continuity of care.

7. Emotional aspects :
It is essential to recognise and respond to the emotional aspects of the transition. Change can be anxiety-provoking for some young adults, especially if they have developed close ties with their paediatric team.

The key to a successful transition is careful planning and preparation, open and ongoing communication between the care teams and the patient, and support and education for the patient to become an active and informed participant in their own care. A well-managed transition can lay the foundations for successful endocrine management in adulthood.

Working with families for optimum care.

Collaboration with families is essential for optimal care, particularly in complex medical fields such as endocrinology. Families play a central role in supporting, understanding and adhering to the care plan, and their active involvement can greatly influence the outcome of treatment.

Understanding family dynamics :
Each family is unique, with its own dynamics, values, beliefs and concerns. A crucial first step is to understand these dynamics. Who makes the decisions? What are the sources of stress or worry within the family? What are their care needs and expectations?

Education and information :
Providing clear, accurate and understandable information is fundamental. Families need to understand the disease, the treatment plan, any side effects, and what they can do to support the patient. The use of brochures, videos, information sessions and workshops can be beneficial.

Active listening :
It is crucial to actively listen to families' concerns and questions. This not only helps us to meet their needs, but also to build a relationship of trust, which is essential for a successful collaboration.

Inclusion in the decision-making process :
Families need to feel involved in decisions about care. This means consulting them, respecting their opinions, and sometimes finding compromises or alternatives that meet both medical needs and family preferences.

Emotional support :
The illness of a loved one can be a source of anxiety, stress and grief for the family. Providing emotional support, whether through counselling, support groups or simply by offering a listening ear, is essential.

Care coordination :
Families can be overwhelmed, especially if they have to coordinate with several specialists or services. Helping with this coordination, for example by providing a single point of contact or arranging consecutive appointments, can ease their burden.

Training and skills :
Sometimes families need to provide care at home, such as administering medication or following a specific diet. In these cases, it is crucial to ensure that they have the necessary skills to do so safely and effectively.

Respect for cultural differences :
Each family may have its own cultural or religious beliefs that influence their perception of the disease and its treatment. It is essential to recognise them, respect them and respond appropriately.

Working with families is an alliance. It requires patience, empathy, communication and a willingness to look beyond the medical aspects to recognise and respond to human needs. When done well, this collaboration can transform care, making the family an active and committed partner in the healing process.

Endocrine disorders specific to paediatrics.

Endocrine pathologies in paediatrics are distinct in many ways from those encountered in adulthood, as they occur at key stages of growth and development. Some of these conditions can have lasting implications, influencing health in adulthood. Here is an overview of common endocrine disorders specific to paediatrics:

1. Growth disorders :
   - **Growth hormone (GH) deficiency**: This condition results from insufficient production of growth hormone, leading to stunted growth.
   - **Congenital adrenal hyperplasia**: can affect growth and sexual development, due to abnormal production of hormones by the adrenal glands.
2. Pubertal disorders :
   - **Precocious puberty**: Puberty begins too early, either in isolation or as a result of abnormal hormone production.
   - **Delayed puberty**: A delay in the onset of puberty, often linked to hormonal problems.
3. Thyroid disorders :
   - **Congenital hypothyroidism**: A thyroid hormone deficiency at birth which, if left untreated, can lead to developmental delays.
   - **Hyperthyroidism**: Although rarer in children, it can occur, often as a result of Graves' disease.

4. Metabolic disorders :

Type 1 diabetes: This is the most common form of diabetes in children and involves autoimmune destruction of the insulin-producing cells in the pancreas.

Neonatal hypoglycaemia: Low blood sugar levels in newborns, which may be due to endocrine causes.

5. Bone and mineral metabolism disorders :

Rickets: Often caused by a vitamin D deficiency, this leads to weak bones in children.

Hyperparathyroidism: Although rare in children, it can occur and affect calcium metabolism.

6. Genetic disorders and syndromes :

Turner syndrome: A genetic disorder affecting girls, often associated with ovarian failure and heart problems.

Klinefelter's syndrome: Affecting boys, it is associated with testicular hypofunction.

7. Adrenal gland disorders :

Congenital adrenal hyperplasia: As mentioned above, this can lead to over- or under-production of certain adrenal hormones.

8. Disorders of sexual development :

Genital ambiguity: The external genitalia do not develop clearly as male or female, often due to hormonal abnormalities.

Treating these conditions requires a multidisciplinary team of paediatric endocrinologists, surgeons, psychologists and other professionals. Early detection and intervention are crucial to ensure optimal outcomes and a better quality of life for the children concerned.

Chapter 7:
ENDOCRINOLOGY AND PREGNANCY

Management of gestational diabetes.

Gestational diabetes (GDM) is a form of diabetes that occurs during pregnancy and affects the way cells use sugar. It can lead to complications for both mother and baby if not managed properly. Here's a fluid, integrated approach to managing gestational diabetes:

The diagnosis of gestational diabetes often comes as a surprise to the mother-to-be. This news, in the midst of the joys and anxieties of pregnancy, can add another layer of worry. However, with appropriate management, most women with GDM can give birth to a healthy baby and return to normal blood sugar levels after delivery.

From the moment of diagnosis, close medical monitoring is essential. Prenatal visits become more frequent, allowing close monitoring of the well-being of both mother and foetus. Self-monitoring of blood sugar levels several times a day quickly becomes routine. These daily measurements provide valuable insight into the body's reactions to food, exercise and other factors.

Diet plays a key role in managing gestational diabetes. A consultation with a dietician can help develop a balanced diet that promotes healthy weight gain during pregnancy while regulating blood sugar levels. Regular meals and snacks, rich in nutrients and low in simple carbohydrates, are often recommended.

Physical activity is another ally. A daily walk, swimming or other forms of exercise adapted to pregnancy can help lower blood sugar levels.

However, for some women, diet and exercise are not enough. In these cases, medication such as insulin may be needed to maintain stable blood sugar levels. The aim is always the same: to protect the mother's health and ensure the baby's optimum development.

Throughout pregnancy, regular ultrasound scans monitor the growth of the foetus. These examinations help to determine whether the baby is growing too quickly, a common concern with gestational diabetes. The date and method of delivery may be influenced by these observations and by blood sugar control.

Once the baby is born, attention turns to the baby and regulating its blood sugar levels. Babies born to mothers who have had GDM may present with hypoglycaemia at birth, which requires monitoring and treatment.

For the mother, monitoring does not stop after childbirth. A post-partum glucose tolerance test is recommended to ensure that blood sugar levels have returned to normal. What's more, women who have developed gestational diabetes have an increased risk of developing type 2 diabetes later in life. So a healthy lifestyle and regular check-ups are essential for prevention.

Managing gestational diabetes is a journey that requires vigilance and commitment, but with the right support, it is entirely possible to get through this period with confidence and optimism for the future of both mother and child.

Thyroid disorders during pregnancy.

Thyroid disorders during pregnancy are conditions that affect the thyroid gland, a small butterfly-shaped gland located at the base of the neck. The thyroid plays a crucial role in regulating metabolism, growth and development. During pregnancy, optimal thyroid function is essential for the health of the mother and the neurological development of the foetus.

1. Hypothyroidism during pregnancy :
Hypothyroidism is a condition in which the thyroid does not produce enough hormones. Symptoms can be subtle and often confused with those typical of pregnancy, such as fatigue, weight gain and depression.

- **Consequences**: If left untreated, hypothyroidism can lead to complications such as foetal growth retardation, premature delivery, pre-eclampsia, low intelligence in the child and even miscarriage.
- **Management**: Screening and treatment with levothyroxine, a synthetic thyroid hormone, are crucial to normalise hormone levels.

2. Hyperthyroidism during pregnancy :
Hyperthyroidism is an excessive production of thyroid hormones. Common causes during pregnancy include Graves' disease and Hashimoto's thyroiditis.

- **Consequences**: Untreated hyperthyroidism can lead to heart failure, heart rhythm disorders, premature delivery, pre-eclampsia, low foetal weight gain, foetal thyroid hyperactivity and, in rare cases, foetal death.
- **Management**: Treatment depends on the cause and severity. Antithyroid drugs, such as propylthiouracil or methimazole, can be used, although their use requires careful monitoring due to potential side effects for the mother and foetus.

3. Goitre during pregnancy :
A goitre is an enlargement of the thyroid gland. It can develop in response to an increased demand for thyroid hormones during pregnancy.

- **Consequences**: A goitre may indicate an underlying problem such as hypothyroidism or hyperthyroidism, but sometimes it may simply be due to iodine deficiency.
- **Management**: The approach depends on the underlying cause. Iodine supplementation may be recommended in cases of deficiency.

4. Post-partum thyroiditis :

This is an inflammation of the thyroid gland that generally occurs a few months after childbirth. It often begins with a phase of hyperthyroidism, followed by hypothyroidism before returning to normal.

- **Consequences**: Symptoms resemble those of the "baby blues" or post-partum depression, such as fatigue, irritability and mood disorders.
- **Management**: Most women recover spontaneously, but some may require treatment, particularly during the hypothyroid phase.

Thyroid function plays an essential role during pregnancy. Thyroid disorders can have serious consequences for both mother and foetus, hence the importance of screening, careful monitoring and appropriate management at every stage of pregnancy.

The importance of endocrine monitoring pre-conception.

Pre-conception endocrine monitoring is an often overlooked but fundamental aspect for women considering pregnancy, particularly those with known endocrine problems or risk factors. The aim of this monitoring is to ensure that the hormonal balance is optimal for conception, foetal development and the smooth progress of the pregnancy. Here are a few reasons why this is so important:

1. Optimising thyroid function :
The thyroid gland has an essential role to play during pregnancy. Sub-optimal thyroid function, whether due to hypothyroidism or hyperthyroidism, can affect fertility and increase the risk of miscarriage, premature delivery, pre-eclampsia and neurodevelopmental disorders in the baby.

2. Diabetes management :
For women with diabetes, whether type 1, type 2 or MODY diabetes, it is crucial to balance blood sugar levels before and during pregnancy. High glucose levels can increase the risk of birth defects, premature delivery and other complications for the baby.

3. Adrenal gland disorders :
Conditions such as congenital adrenal hyperplasia must be carefully managed before conception to ensure that both mother and foetus have an appropriate hormonal balance, minimising the risk of complications.

4. Hyperprolactinaemia :
High prolactin levels can interfere with ovulation and therefore fertility. Identifying and treating the cause can increase the chances of conceiving naturally.

5. Ovulation disorders linked to hormones :
Polycystic ovary syndrome (PCOS) is a common cause of infertility linked to hormonal imbalance. Endocrine management can help regulate menstrual cycles and improve the chances of conception.

6. Medication and pregnancy :
Certain medications used to treat endocrine disorders are not safe during pregnancy. An endocrinologist can help to

adjust or change treatments before conception to ensure that they are safe for the developing foetus.

7. Prevention of complications :
Endocrine monitoring allows potential risks to be identified and managed before they become a problem during pregnancy, thus preventing complications that could harm the mother or child.

8. Education and advice :
This follow-up is also an opportunity to educate mothers-to-be about the importance of hormonal balance during pregnancy, the implications of their endocrine conditions, and the steps they can take to ensure a healthy pregnancy. Pre-conception endocrine monitoring is an essential part of family planning for many women. It lays the foundations for a healthy pregnancy by ensuring that conditions are optimal for conception and foetal development, while enabling potential risks to be prevented and managed proactively.

Post-partum support and breastfeeding.

Post-partum care is a crucial stage for both mother and child, and endocrinology-related issues play a significant role, particularly in the context of breastfeeding. This delicate stage in a woman's life, commonly referred to as the 'fourth trimester', requires special attention to ensure the physical and emotional well-being of the mother and to promote the healthy development of the baby.

1. The importance of hormones in breastfeeding :
Breastfeeding is a process that is strongly regulated by hormones, mainly prolactin and oxytocin. These hormones not only trigger the production and expulsion of milk, but

also have an impact on the mother's mood and emotional well-being.

2. Post-partum endocrine challenges :
   Post-partum thyroiditis: This is an inflammation of the thyroid gland that can lead to hyperthyroidism followed by hypothyroidism. It can affect mood and energy, essential aspects of adjusting to life with a newborn.

   Adrenal gland dysfunction: The stress of childbirth, coupled with sleep deprivation, can affect the adrenal glands, impacting on the mother's ability to cope with stress.

3. Breastfeeding support :
   Medication and breastfeeding: Some women may require medication for endocrine conditions. It is crucial to ensure that these medications are compatible with breastfeeding.

   Endocrinology-related breastfeeding problems: Endocrine disorders, such as PCOS or certain thyroid conditions, can influence lactation. Specialist support may be required for these women.

4. Emotional and psychological aspects :
Post-partum hormonal balance can greatly influence mood and emotional well-being. Hormones, coupled with the physical and emotional challenges of caring for a newborn, can make some women more vulnerable to disorders such as post-partum depression.

5. Advice and education :
It is essential to inform and advise new mothers about the hormonal changes they may experience, how these changes may affect their ability to breastfeed, and how to manage them.

6. Medical follow-up :
Regular medical check-ups with an endocrinologist can be beneficial for women with a history of endocrine disorders or post-partum symptoms. This allows any hormonal imbalance to be identified and treated quickly.

7. Multidisciplinary collaboration :
Post-partum support and breastfeeding may require collaboration between several professionals: endocrinologists, obstetricians, paediatricians, midwives, lactation consultants and therapists or psychologists specialising in post-partum mental health.

The post-partum period is one of profound physical and emotional change, influenced by a cascade of hormonal fluctuations. Appropriate support, focused on the mother's endocrine well-being, is fundamental to ensuring a healthy transition to this new phase of life, promoting the mother's well-being and the baby's optimal health.

Chapter 8:
GERIATRIC ENDOCRINOLOGY

Endocrine changes with age.

The endocrine system, which encompasses all the glands and hormones in our body, plays a crucial role in regulating many vital functions. As we age, this system, like many other aspects of our physiology, undergoes significant changes. Understanding these changes can help us to anticipate and manage some of the challenges associated with ageing.

1. Thyroid function :
   - With age, it is common to see a slight increase in TSH (thyroid stimulating hormone), although thyroid hormone levels remain within the normal range.
   - The risk of hypothyroidism, where the thyroid gland does not produce enough hormones, increases with age. Similarly, thyroid nodules are more common in older people.
2. Sex hormones :
   - **For women**: The menopause, generally around the age of 50, marks the end of reproduction. It is characterised by a significant drop in oestrogen and progesterone levels.
   - **In men**: Although there is no equivalent male 'menopause', there is a progressive decline in testosterone with age, sometimes referred to as andropause. This decline can be associated with symptoms such as fatigue, reduced libido, loss of muscle mass and mood changes.

3. Insulin and glucose homeostasis :
   - Insulin resistance tends to increase with age, which means that the body needs more insulin to effectively regulate blood sugar levels.
   - This increase in insulin resistance is one of the reasons why the risk of developing type 2 diabetes increases with age.
4. Growth hormones and insulin-like growth factor (IGF-1) :
   - Growth hormone secretion decreases significantly with age, leading to a drop in IGF-1 levels. This can contribute to a loss of muscle mass and an increase in fat mass.
5. Adrenal hormones :
   - Production of DHEA and its sulphated form (DHEA-S), hormone precursors produced by the adrenal glands, declines with age. It is thought that this decline may play a role in ageing and chronic disease.
   - The ability of the adrenal glands to produce cortisol in response to stress can also decline with age.
6. Parathyroid hormone and bone metabolism :
   - With age, intestinal calcium absorption decreases, and vitamin D levels may also fall. In response, parathyroid hormone (PTH) rises, increasing the risk of osteoporosis and fractures.
7. Antidiuretic hormone (ADH) :
   - The ability to concentrate urine decreases with age, partly due to changes in ADH production and response. This can increase the risk of dehydration in the elderly.

In short, ageing is accompanied by a series of endocrine changes that can have significant consequences for health and well-being. A thorough understanding of these changes, together with regular monitoring and appropriate interventions, can help us to navigate the challenges of ageing more serenely.

Management of endocrine diseases in the elderly patient.

Managing endocrine diseases in the elderly patient is a particular challenge because of the co-morbidities often present, the physiological changes associated with age and the particular implications of these diseases for older people. The following is a holistic approach to the management of endocrine diseases in the elderly patient:

1. Hypothyroidism :
   - In the elderly, symptoms may be atypical (such as lethargy, confusion, intolerance to cold or even depression).
   - When starting treatment, it is advisable to start with a low dose of levothyroxine and adjust gradually to avoid undesirable cardiac effects.
2. Hyperthyroidism :
   - Symptoms may be less pronounced in the elderly, but the risk of arrhythmia, particularly atrial fibrillation, is higher.
   - Synthetic antithyroid drugs or treatment with radioactive iodine may be considered depending on the severity and cause.
3. Diabetes :
   - Diabetes management in elderly patients must be individualised, taking into account the risk of hypoglycaemia, co-morbidities and life expectancy.
   - Glycaemic targets can be relaxed to avoid hypoglycaemia, especially in patients with a history of falls or cognitive impairment.
4. Osteoporosis :
   - Regular assessment of bone density can help determine the risk of fracture.
   - Calcium and vitamin D supplementation, combined with bisphosphonates or other drugs, may be recommended to reduce the risk.

5. Adrenal adenomas :
   - These tumours are frequently detected by chance in the elderly. Their functionality needs to be assessed and their size monitored.
   - Non-functional adenomas that remain stable in size can simply be monitored, while those that secrete hormones or increase in size may require intervention.
6. Hypogonadism :
   - The decline in testosterone in older men (sometimes called andropause) must be distinguished from normal ageing.
   - Testosterone supplementation is controversial and should be considered on a case-by-case basis, assessing the potential benefits and risks (particularly cardiovascular).
7. Drug monitoring :
   - The elderly are often polimedicated, which increases the risk of drug interactions.
   - It is essential to regularly reassess medications, particularly those used to treat endocrine disorders, and to adjust doses if necessary.

8. Multidisciplinary approach :
   - The management of endocrine diseases in elderly patients often requires collaboration between endocrinologists, geriatricians, cardiologists, nephrologists and other specialists.
   - Collaboration with dieticians, physiotherapists and social workers can also be beneficial.
9. Education and communication :
   - It is crucial to educate elderly patients and their carers about their endocrine disorders, providing them with clear and appropriate information.
10. Taking quality of life into account :
   - Beyond the figures and diagnoses, it is essential to take account of the patient's quality of life, preferences and values when making therapeutic decisions.

The management of endocrine diseases in elderly patients requires an individualised approach, taking into account the complexity of the medical, psychological and social challenges specific to this population. Open communication, appropriate education and multidisciplinary management are essential to ensure optimal treatment and improve quality of life.

Importance of polypharmacy and drug interactions.

Polypharmacy, which refers to the simultaneous use of several medicines by a patient, is a growing concern in medicine, particularly among elderly patients or those with multiple pathologies. While it is sometimes necessary to manage complex conditions, polypharmacy can also entail a series of challenges and risks. One of the major problems associated with polypharmacy is the potential for drug interactions. Here's an exploration of the importance of polypharmacy and drug interactions:

1. Increased risk of side effects :
Each drug has its own side-effect profile. When several drugs are combined, the risk of experiencing one or more of these side effects may increase.

2. Drug interactions :
- **Pharmacodynamic interaction**: This occurs when two or more drugs have additive or antagonistic effects. For example, if two drugs lower blood pressure, their combined effect could cause dangerous hypotension.
- **Pharmacokinetic interaction**: This occurs when one drug affects the absorption, distribution, metabolism or elimination of another drug. For example, one drug

may inhibit a liver enzyme that metabolises another drug, leading to higher levels of the latter in the blood.

3. Medication non-compliance :
With a large number of medicines to take, the patient's ability to follow the prescribed regimen correctly can diminish, leading to omissions, double doses or other errors.

4. Increased risk of falls :
Several drugs, particularly those that affect the central nervous system (such as sedatives or antihypertensives), can increase the risk of falls in the elderly.

5. High costs :
Polypharmacy can lead to considerable drug costs for patients and the healthcare system.

6. Risk of cascade prescriptions :
This is when the side effects of a drug are misinterpreted as a new condition, leading to the prescription of other drugs, thus exacerbating polypharmacy.

7. Follow-up difficulties :
With many drugs, keeping track of doses, schedules and potential interactions can become complex for carers and healthcare professionals.

Strategies for managing polypharmacy :
- **Regular review of medicines**: It is essential to regularly review all the medicines a patient is taking, assessing the need for and effectiveness of each.
- **Prioritise medicines**: Whenever possible, give priority to essential drugs and consider de-escalating or stopping non-essential drugs.
- **Education**: Ensuring that patients and their carers understand the purpose of each drug, how to take it correctly, and are aware of potential side effects.

Use tools and technologies: Pillboxes, reminder apps and other tools can help patients manage their medication effectively.

Although polypharmacy may be necessary in some cases, it requires careful attention and monitoring to minimise the risks and maximise the benefits. Recognising the importance of drug interactions and adopting a patient-centred approach can greatly improve the quality of care and patient safety.

Supporting quality of life and autonomy.

Quality of life and independence are key objectives in the care of all individuals, particularly the elderly, patients with chronic illnesses and people with disabilities. Promoting a good quality of life and supporting independence involves a holistic approach that takes into account the physical, psychological, social and emotional needs of each individual. Here are some key elements to consider in this process:

1. Overall assessment :
    Functional assessment: This involves examining the person's ability to carry out essential daily activities such as feeding, dressing and washing, as well as more complex tasks such as shopping or managing finances.

    Psychological assessment: Identify any signs of depression, anxiety or other mental health problems that could affect quality of life.
2. Appropriate medical management :
    Minimise polypharmacy where possible and manage medicines to avoid side effects or interactions that could affect mobility or cognition.

Regular monitoring to manage chronic conditions and prevent complications.

3. Physiotherapy and rehabilitation :
- Appropriate exercises can help improve strength, balance and mobility, reducing the risk of falls and promoting independence.
- Rehabilitation can be essential after events such as a stroke or surgery.

4. Psychological and social support :
- Offer access to therapies or support groups.
- Encouraging socialisation to combat isolation, whether through group activities, clubs or community events.

5. Technical aids and home improvements :
- Devices such as walking sticks, walkers, stairlifts or grab rails can help maintain independence in the home.
- Adapting the home to make it accessible and safe: for example, removing obstacles, installing ramps, widening doors for wheelchairs, etc.

6. Education and training :
- Educating people about their condition, the medication they are taking and the strategies they can use to maintain or improve their quality of life.
- For patients with chronic illnesses, such as diabetes, offer training on how to manage their disease.

7. Support for carers :
- Carers play a crucial role in maintaining people's quality of life and independence, so it's essential to support them, provide them with resources and, if necessary, give them a break (respite care).

8. Encouraging self-efficacy :
- Helping individuals to recognise their abilities and develop skills to manage their health and well-being can boost their confidence and autonomy.

9. Integrating individual preferences and values :
- Shared decision-making, which takes account of each individual's wishes, values and preferences, is

essential to ensure that care is in line with what is most important to them.

Supporting quality of life and independence is a multi-dimensional endeavour that requires an integrated, individualised and person-centred approach. The key lies in understanding the unique needs of each individual and putting in place appropriate strategies to support them in their journey towards health and well-being.

Chapter 9:
TECHNOLOGY AND TELEMEDICINE IN ENDOCRINOLOGY

The use of insulin pumps and continuous glucose monitors.

Developments in medical technology have led to significant advances in the management of diabetes, particularly with the development of insulin pumps and continuous glucose monitors (CGMs). Used alone or in combination, these tools can considerably improve diabetes management and patients' quality of life.

1. Insulin pumps :

   What is an insulin pump? An insulin pump is an electronic device the size of a small mobile phone that delivers insulin continuously 24 hours a day. It replaces the need for multiple daily injections of insulin.

   Benefits: Pumps can improve glycaemic control by allowing more precise and flexible adjustments to insulin doses. They can reduce extreme variations in blood sugar levels, lower the risk of nocturnal hypoglycaemia and offer greater flexibility in daily routines.

   Considerations: Using a pump requires training, careful monitoring and regular adjustments. It is often recommended for patients who have difficulty maintaining good glycaemic control with injections.

2. Continuous glucose monitors (CGMs) :

   What is a CGM? A CGM is a device that measures blood glucose levels continuously throughout the day and night. It consists of a sensor inserted under the skin that measures glucose levels in the interstitial fluid (the fluid around the cells).

Benefits: GCMs provide a detailed view of blood glucose variations, enabling patients and healthcare providers to adjust treatment accordingly. They can alert patients to impending hypoglycaemia or hyperglycaemia, which can be particularly useful at night or in patients who do not feel the symptoms of hypoglycaemia.

Considerations: As with pumps, using a GCM requires training. Some GCMs also require calibration with a conventional glucose meter.

3. Integrated systems - insulin pumps and MCGs :

Some systems combine the insulin pump and the MCG to provide a 'closed loop' or artificial pancreas system. This means that the MCG communicates directly with the pump to adjust insulin delivery according to glucose readings, reducing the need for manual intervention.

These systems can significantly improve glycaemic control, reduce the risk of hypo- and hyperglycaemic episodes and offer patients and their families greater peace of mind.

4. Factors to consider :

Patient choice: While these technologies offer many advantages, they are not suitable for everyone. The choice to use them should be based on individual preferences, lifestyle, age, adherence to treatment and ability to manage the technology.

Costs and insurance cover: Pumps and GCMs can be expensive, so it's essential to look at the insurance cover and assistance programmes available.

Education and support: Thorough training and ongoing support are essential if these devices are to be used effectively.

Insulin pumps and CGMs have revolutionised diabetes management, providing patients with tools that can significantly improve glycaemic control and quality of life. As with all medical decisions, it is essential to adopt a patient-centred approach, weighing up the pros and cons according to individual needs and preferences.

Remote consultations and virtual patient follow-up.

Telemedicine, which encompasses remote consultations and the virtual monitoring of patients, has grown in popularity in recent years, not least because of technological advances and global circumstances such as the COVID-19 pandemic. It offers greater flexibility, improves access to care and can reduce the costs associated with face-to-face consultations. However, there are also challenges associated with its use. Let's take a look at the benefits, limitations and implications of this care modality.

Advantages :
- **Accessibility**: Telemedicine can eliminate geographical barriers, enabling patients living in rural or remote areas to access specialists and care without having to travel.
- **Flexibility**: consultations can be scheduled outside traditional office hours, which suits many patients and healthcare professionals.
- **Cost savings**: Patients can save money and time by avoiding travel. It can also reduce costs for healthcare establishments by minimising the use of infrastructure.
- **Continuity of care**: Telemedicine can facilitate regular monitoring, particularly for patients with chronic illnesses.

- **Safety**: During epidemics or emergency situations, telemedicine can reduce the risk of exposure while guaranteeing continuity of care.

Limits :

- **Technological limitations**: Not all patients have access to a stable Internet connection or to the devices needed for remote consultations.
- **Technological skills**: Some patients, particularly the elderly, may be uncomfortable with technology or have difficulty using it.
- **Quality of care**: Some conditions require a physical examination or other interventions that cannot be performed virtually.
- **Confidentiality and security**: It is crucial to ensure that telemedicine platforms comply with patient data confidentiality and security standards.

Implications for practice :

- **Training and education**: Healthcare professionals need to be trained in the use of technology and how to conduct effective remote consultations.
- **Informed consent**: It is essential to inform patients of the benefits and limits of telemedicine and to obtain their consent.
- **Integration with traditional care**: Telemedicine must be seamlessly integrated into the patient's overall care pathway, in collaboration with face-to-face care.
- **Adaptability**: Professionals must be prepared to adapt, whether to manage technological problems or to identify situations where face-to-face consultation is necessary.

Telemedicine has the potential to transform the way care is delivered, making medicine more accessible, efficient and patient-centred. However, to maximise the benefits, it is essential to proactively address the challenges and ensure that the technology is used in a way that complements traditional care, while focusing on the quality, safety and integrity of care.

The importance of technological training for nurses.

In the age of digitisation and cutting-edge medicine, technology plays an essential role in almost every aspect of healthcare. For nurses, professionals on the front line of care, adapting to this technological wave is not only beneficial but crucial. Here's why technology training is of paramount importance for nurses:

1. Improving precision and efficiency :
The use of electronic medical records (EMRs) and other digital tools can reduce manual errors, ensure rapid access to patient information and facilitate the coordination of care between different healthcare professionals.

2. Real-time monitoring and intervention :
Many modern medical devices, from heart monitors to infusion pumps, are now connected and can transmit data in real time. Nurses trained in these technologies can react quickly to changes in a patient's condition.

3. Telemedicine and remote care :
With the rise of telemedicine, nurses can play a key role in providing remote care, whether for patient monitoring, education or initial consultations.

4. Access to educational and professional resources
Technology gives nurses access to a multitude of educational resources, from webinars to online courses, enabling them to keep up to date with the latest practices and research.

5. Improved communication :
Digital communication platforms encourage better collaboration between care teams, whether to discuss a patient's care, transfer responsibilities or consult on complex cases.

6. Security and confidentiality :
Appropriate training enables nurses to understand the importance of data security and confidentiality, and to take appropriate measures to protect sensitive patient information.

7. Patient empowerment :
Many patients now use apps and devices to monitor their health. Technologically trained nurses can help patients navigate these tools and use them effectively.

8. Workload management :
Technological solutions, such as patient management systems or scheduling applications, can help nurses to manage their workload, prioritise tasks and ensure optimum attention for each patient.

9. Adaptability in the face of a rapidly changing medical landscape :
Medical technology is evolving rapidly. To remain relevant and effective in their role, nurses must be ready to adopt new solutions as they emerge.

Technological training is not just an asset; it has become a necessity for nurses. In an ever-changing medical world, equipping nurses with the skills they need to competently navigate today's technological environment not only ensures better quality care, but also reinforces the essential role of nurses as pillars of the healthcare system.

Telemedicine as
a tool for interdisciplinary collaboration.

Telemedicine has evolved considerably, from a simple means of remote consultation to a dynamic collaborative platform for healthcare professionals from a variety of disciplines. It is now an essential tool for effective interdisciplinary collaboration, promoting an integrated approach to care. Here's how telemedicine facilitates this collaboration:

1. Greater access to a wide range of experts :
Telemedicine enables teams of doctors, nurses, pharmacists, therapists and other healthcare professionals to work together, regardless of their geographical location. This is particularly valuable for rural or underserved areas, where certain specialities may be absent.

2. Joint real-time consultations :
Experts in different fields can consult simultaneously on a complex case, enabling informed decision-making. For example, a cardiologist, a nephrologist and a general practitioner can discuss the best treatment options for a patient together.

3. Coordinated patient follow-up :
Telemedicine facilitates the coordinated monitoring of patients across different specialities, ensuring that all the professionals involved are up to date with the latest developments, treatments and care plans.

4. Interprofessional education and training :
Healthcare professionals can work together to offer seminars, workshops and training to their peers, sharing knowledge and best practice across different disciplines.

5. Interdisciplinary case reviews :
Telemedicine enables teams to discuss cases regularly, share perspectives and formulate care recommendations collectively.

6. Sharing resources and information :
The technology integrated into telemedicine facilitates the sharing of medical records, diagnostic images and other relevant information between professionals, which is essential for holistic patient care.

7. Improving communication :
Communication is central to interdisciplinary collaboration. Telemedicine offers platforms that enable fluid and efficient communication, reducing misunderstandings and overlaps.

8. Patient-centred care :
Interdisciplinary collaboration via telemedicine ensures that the patient is at the heart of the discussions, with an integrated approach that takes account of all aspects of his or her health.

9. Cost and efficiency savings :
Coordination via telemedicine can reduce the need for patients to make multiple visits to different specialists, thereby minimising travel, costs and time.

10. Flexibility :
The ability to organise virtual meetings and consultations offers unprecedented flexibility to professionals, enabling them to work together at times that suit their constraints.

As a tool for interdisciplinary collaboration, telemedicine is transforming the way healthcare professionals interact, learn and care for patients. It promotes an integrated approach to care, ensuring that each patient benefits from collective expertise for optimal outcomes. As technology continues to evolve, it is likely that the impact of telemedicine on interdisciplinary collaboration will only increase.

Chapter 10:
PSYCHOSOCIAL ASPECTS
IN ENDOCRINOLOGY

Understanding the emotional impact endocrine diseases.

Endocrine diseases, like other medical conditions, can have a profound impact on a person's emotional and psychological well-being. Understanding these impacts is essential, not only for the patient themselves, but also for carers, family and friends, in order to provide appropriate support and facilitate disease management.

Hormonal imbalances, at the heart of endocrine disorders, have a direct influence on mood, cognition and behaviour. For example, thyroid fluctuations can trigger feelings of anxiety, depression or irritability. Similarly, people with diabetes may experience stress or anxiety linked to the constant management of their blood sugar levels, the fear of complications or the sheer pressure of having to live with a chronic disease.

Add to this the burden of physical symptoms - fatigue, weight changes, changes in body appearance - which can lead to feelings of insecurity, social isolation or low self-esteem. The emotional implications of endocrine diseases can also have a domino effect on relationships, work and general quality of life. Patients may feel misunderstood or stigmatised, especially if their symptoms are not immediately apparent to others.

It is crucial to recognise that these emotional reactions are not simply 'side-effects' of the disease, but are an intrinsic part of the patient's experience. The approach to care must therefore be holistic, taking into account both physiological and psychological needs.

Healthcare professionals need to be trained to recognise the signs of emotional distress and direct patients to appropriate resources, whether these be support groups, therapy or other interventions. Patients, for their part, can benefit from learning coping strategies, practising mindfulness or simply sharing their feelings with others who are going through similar experiences.

Understanding the emotional impact of endocrine diseases is an essential step in providing comprehensive and compassionate care. Each patient is a complex, multifaceted entity, and their emotional well-being is intimately linked to their physical health.

Specific psychological support: depression, anxiety, body image disorders.

Psychological support for patients with endocrine diseases is essential. The manifestation and management of these diseases can often lead to feelings of depression, anxiety and body image disorders. Each of these aspects deserves special attention to ensure holistic patient care.

Depression:
Depression can be both a consequence and an aggravating factor of endocrine diseases. Hormonal imbalance can influence brain chemistry and affect mood, leading to persistent feelings of sadness, disinterest or hopelessness. In addition, the daily challenges of managing a chronic illness can weigh heavily on the mind, exacerbating feelings of depression. Therapeutic support, whether in the form of individual therapy, antidepressant

medication or support groups, is essential to help patients navigate these troubled waters and return to a balanced and fulfilling life.

Anxiety :

The uncertainty associated with the progression of the disease, the results of medical tests or potential complications can be a major source of anxiety. In addition, certain hormonal imbalances can directly cause anxiety symptoms. Early recognition of these symptoms is crucial. Techniques such as cognitive behavioural therapy, meditation or guided breathing **can be used to manage anxiety.**

Body image disorders :

Endocrine diseases, such as thyroid disorders or polycystic ovary syndrome, can lead to noticeable physical changes, such as weight gain or loss, hair loss or skin problems. These changes can have a profound effect on a person's self-perception and self-esteem. Psychological support, often in the form of individual therapy or support groups, can help patients rebuild their self-image and develop positive acceptance and appreciation of their bodies.

An essential factor to remember is that the body and mind are intrinsically linked. An imbalance or disturbance in one can have repercussions on the other. Specific psychological support must therefore be seen not as a secondary consideration, but as an integral part of the patient's overall care. By recognising and addressing these psychological aspects, we can not only improve patients' quality of life but also potentially improve their medical outcomes.

Support for specific groups: teenagers, transgender people, infertility patients.

The management of endocrine diseases requires special attention for specific groups who may face unique challenges because of their situation or identity. Adolescents, transgender people and infertile patients, for example, may have specific emotional and psychological needs that merit tailored care.

Teenagers :
Adolescence is a time of transition, rapid growth and significant hormonal changes. Adolescents with endocrine diseases can face challenges such as stigma from peers, low self-esteem or difficulties adhering to treatment. Age-appropriate support can include:
- Consultations with psychologists specialising in adolescent issues.
- Setting up support groups for teenagers facing similar challenges.
- Education on disease management at a time when independence and responsibility are on the increase.

Transgender people :
Transgender people seeking to align their gender identity with their body may resort to hormone treatments. These treatments, while essential for their well-being, can also entail emotional and physiological challenges.
- Psychological support to help you cope with body changes and societal reactions.
- Clear information and education on the effects and implications of hormone treatments.
- Support groups or communities where you can share experiences and advice.

Infertile patients :
Infertility can have profound emotional repercussions, often accompanied by feelings of loss, shame or guilt. Couples or individuals concerned may need :

- Individual or couple therapy to deal with grief, stress or relationship tensions linked to infertility.
- Support groups where you can share experiences and get advice.
- Education about the options available, whether medical treatment or other avenues such as adoption or surrogate motherhood.

The management of endocrine diseases goes far beyond medical treatment. For the specific groups mentioned, emotional and psychological support is essential to ensure optimal quality of life and lasting well-being. It is imperative for healthcare professionals to adopt a holistic approach, taking into account the individual and unique needs of each patient and offering care tailored to those needs.

Communication techniques to tackle sensitive subjects.

Discussing sensitive issues with patients or their families requires empathetic, thoughtful and respectful communication. These delicate moments may be linked to a difficult diagnosis, complex treatment decisions or unexpected news. Here are some communication techniques that can facilitate these delicate discussions while respecting the feelings and concerns of those involved:

1. Creating the right environment :
Choose a quiet, private place for the conversation. Make sure the setting is comfortable for all parties and avoid potential interruptions.

2. Active listening :
Pay full attention to what the patient or family is saying. This means listening not only with your ears, but also with your heart and mind. Note their concerns, hesitations and feelings.

3. Use simple, clear language:
Avoid medical or technical jargon. Express yourself concisely and make sure the information is clearly understood.

4. Validating emotions :
Acknowledge and validate the patient's or family's feelings. Phrases such as "I understand why you might feel that way" or "It's perfectly normal to feel that way" can be comforting.

5. Ask open-ended questions:
Questions such as "How do you feel about this?" or "What are your main concerns?" can encourage dialogue and give patients the opportunity to express their feelings.

6. Show empathy:
Show that you really care about the patient's feelings and concerns. A simple statement such as "I'm really sorry you're going through this" can have a significant impact.

7. Be patient:
Give the patient or family time to process the information, and be prepared to repeat or clarify if necessary.

8. Offer support :
Refer the patient or family to additional resources, whether support groups, therapy or other health professionals.

9. Involve the patient in the decision-making process :
Make patients feel that they have a voice in decisions about their care. This can help them feel more in control and reduce anxiety or fear.

10. Practise emotional regulation:
It is crucial for healthcare professionals to manage their own emotions during sensitive discussions in order to remain focused and present for the patient.

11. Ask for feedback :
After sharing information, ask the patient or family if they have any questions or if there is anything they haven't understood.

12. Conclude with concrete steps:
End the conversation by summarising the main points raised and discussing the next steps or actions to be taken.

In all exchanges, respect, compassion and honesty must be at the heart of communication. By adopting an empathetic, patient-centred approach, healthcare professionals can address sensitive issues in a respectful and constructive way, while building trust and mutual support.

Chapter 11:
NUTRITION AND ENDOCRINOLOGY

Basic principles of nutrition in endocrinology.

Nutrition plays an essential role in endocrinology, as hormones regulate many of the body's metabolic functions, influencing the absorption, distribution and use of nutrients. Adopting an appropriate diet can help to manage, prevent or even reverse certain endocrine disorders.

The balance between carbohydrates, proteins and fats is crucial, particularly for people with diabetes, a condition in which insulin, a hormone produced by the pancreas, does not work properly. Precise control of carbohydrate intake, in conjunction with medication or insulin, is essential to maintain stable blood glucose levels.

Similarly, people with thyroid disorders, whether hypo- or hyperthyroid, need to watch what they eat. Underweight or overweight can affect the secretion of thyroid hormones, and certain nutrients, such as iodine, are essential for the synthesis of these hormones.

For patients with polycystic ovary syndrome (PCOS), a common endocrine disorder in women of childbearing age, a suitable diet can help manage symptoms. PCOS is often associated with insulin resistance, and a diet low in carbohydrates can be beneficial.

In addition, parathyroid hormones regulate calcium levels in the blood, and a diet rich in calcium, combined with vitamin D, is recommended for people suffering from hypoparathyroidism, where there is insufficient production of these hormones.

Nutrition in endocrinology therefore goes far beyond simple diet. It is deeply intertwined with the body's biochemistry, affected by and in turn influencing the hormones that regulate so many bodily functions. Each endocrine condition may require a slightly different nutritional approach, and working closely with specialist dieticians and endocrinologists is essential to ensure that patients receive not only the nutrients they need, but also the education and support they need to proactively manage their condition.

Specific dietetics :
Diabetes, thyroid disorders, obesity.

Dietetics is a fundamental pillar in the management of many endocrine conditions, including diabetes, thyroid disorders and obesity. Each condition presents its own challenges and requires a tailored nutritional approach to ensure optimal disease management.

Diabetes :
Managing diabetes revolves mainly around regulating blood sugar levels. Key elements include:
- **Carbohydrate control**: Monitoring carbohydrate intake and understanding its impact on blood glucose levels is essential. This can be managed through meal planning and, in some cases, by using techniques such as carbohydrate counting.
- **Foods with a low glycaemic index (GI)**: These foods cause a slower, more stable rise in blood sugar levels.
- **Dietary fibre**: Can help regulate blood sugar peaks and improve insulin sensitivity.

Thyroid disorders:

Diet can play a role in the management of thyroid disorders, although recommendations vary depending on the specific nature of the disorder.

- **Iodine**: This is a key element in the production of thyroid hormones. A balanced diet with appropriate sources of iodine (such as seafood and iodised salt) is essential.
- **Avoidance of goitrogens**: In some cases, it may be advisable to limit consumption of goitrogenic foods (such as soya, kale and broccoli), especially if you are iodine-deficient.

Obesity :

Obesity is often linked to endocrine imbalances and insulin resistance. A dietary approach to managing obesity could include:

- **Calorie deficit**: This is essential for weight loss. It means consuming fewer calories than your body expends.
- **Protein**: A diet rich in protein can help you feel full and maintain muscle mass during weight loss.
- **Reducing simple sugars and saturated fats**: Opting for sources of complex carbohydrates and healthy fats can improve the quality of your diet and support weight loss.
- **Hydration**: Drinking enough water can help with satiety and elimination.

It is crucial to note that, while diet is a key element in the management of these endocrine disorders, it is only one part of the equation. A holistic approach that includes exercise, appropriate medication and psychological support is often necessary for effective management. What's more, each individual is unique; what works for one person may not work for another. It is therefore essential to work closely with healthcare professionals to develop a plan tailored to each individual.

Working with nutritionists/dieticians.

Collaboration between endocrinology professionals and nutritionists or dieticians is crucial to ensuring optimal care for patients suffering from endocrine diseases. Their joint expertise enables comprehensive, personalised treatment plans to be drawn up, combining in-depth nutritional advice with medical management of hormonal disorders.

1. Integrated approach to care :
A patient with endocrine disease, whether diabetes, thyroid disorders or obesity, often requires specific nutritional advice. The endocrinologist, while an expert in hormones, may not have the time or detailed expertise to provide in-depth dietary advice. This is where the dietician comes in, providing expertise on foods, portions, food substitutions and specific diets.

2. Education and training :
Nutritionists and dieticians can provide targeted nutritional education, helping patients to understand how their food choices affect their endocrine condition. They can organise workshops, information sessions and individual consultations to educate and advise patients.

3. Personalised meal plans :
Every patient is unique, with their own nutritional needs, food preferences and lifestyle. Dietitians work closely with patients to develop meal plans that are tailored to their medical condition, yet achievable and enjoyable.

4. Follow-up and adjustments :
Nutrition is dynamic, and what works for a patient at one point may need to be adjusted later. Dietitians provide regular monitoring, assessing progress, identifying obstacles and making changes to the diet plan if necessary.

5. Search and update :
The field of nutrition is constantly evolving, with new research and discoveries emerging. Dietitians keep up to date with the latest advances and can incorporate this knowledge into the advice they give, ensuring that patients benefit from the best recommendations available.

6. Emotional support and motivation :
Dietary changes can be difficult. Dietitians often offer emotional support, encourage patients, help them overcome obstacles and motivate them to pursue their nutritional goals.
The collaboration between endocrinologists and nutritionists/dietitians is a powerful synergy, combining medical and nutritional expertise for the optimum benefit of patients. Together, they can offer holistic, patient-centred care that addresses not only the medical needs, but also the dietary, emotional and lifestyle needs of patients.

Patient education food self-management.

Patient education in dietary self-management is an essential part of the management of endocrine disorders. This is particularly crucial for diseases such as diabetes, where food choices have a direct impact on blood glucose levels. Here's how it can be approached in a fluid and comprehensive way:

Food self-management is not just about the food we eat. It's about instilling a deep understanding of the interactions between food, metabolism and medication. It encompasses the knowledge, skills and confidence to make food choices that support wellbeing while effectively managing illness.

Firstly, it is crucial to demystify the basic concepts of nutrition, by clarifying the roles of the macronutrients - carbohydrates, proteins and fats. For a diabetic patient, for example, this would mean understanding how carbohydrates affect blood sugar levels, how protein can stabilise this response, and how fats, although necessary, should be consumed with discernment.

But knowing the facts is not enough. It's essential to adapt this knowledge to everyday life. This could mean learning to read and interpret nutrition labels, identifying foods rich in hidden carbohydrates, or even planning balanced meals. A trip to the supermarket can turn into an educational session, choosing foods that align with dietary needs while balancing preferences and budgetary constraints.

Challenges can arise in social situations, such as restaurant meals or family gatherings. Here, the emphasis is on strategy: how to make intelligent choices from a menu, how to balance occasional indulgences with the daily routine, or how to deal with peer pressure or cultural traditions.

Technology is also playing an increasing role in dietary self-management. From food tracking apps to gadgets that analyse the composition of meals, technological equipment can be a valuable tool in helping patients stay on track.

But at the heart of it all, there is a human component. Self-management of food can be emotionally charged, linked to feelings of deprivation, frustration or shame. Psychological support, whether in the form of individual therapy, support groups or simply empathetic education sessions, is fundamental.

Food self-management education aims to empower patients. With the right skills and support, they can navigate the complex world of nutrition with confidence, making choices that not only support their health, but also enrich their lives.

Chapter 12:
ENDOCRINOLOGY AND SPORT

Managing diabetes in athletes.

Managing diabetes in sport is a complex balancing act, requiring particular attention to energy requirements, variations in blood glucose levels, adaptation of treatment and monitoring. Physical activities, whether endurance, strength or team sports, have a considerable impact on the metabolism, and consequently on the insulin and carbohydrate requirements, of diabetic athletes.

Assessment and planning :
Before starting an exercise programme or taking part in a sporting competition, diabetic athletes should consult their medical team. A prior assessment of insulin requirements, eating habits and the type of exercise planned will help to draw up a suitable action plan.

Monitoring blood glucose levels :
It is vital for diabetic athletes to monitor their blood sugar levels frequently before, during and after exercise. This allows them to adjust their carbohydrate intake and treatment according to their needs. Continuous glucose monitors (CGM) can be particularly useful for tracking trends and anticipating needs.

Carbohydrate intake :
Exercise increases insulin sensitivity, which can lead to a drop in blood sugar levels. It is essential to compensate for this drop with an adequate carbohydrate intake before, during and after exercise. Specific needs will vary according to the intensity and duration of exercise.

Insulin adjustment :
Depending on the type, duration and intensity of the activity, athletes may need to reduce their insulin dose to avoid hypoglycaemia. Insulin pumps allow flexible adjustments and can be particularly useful for diabetic athletes.

Complication management :
It is essential to recognise and treat signs of hypoglycaemia quickly, such as shaking, sweating or confusion. Having quick sources of glucose, such as energy gels or sweets, on hand at all times is crucial.

Recovery and rest:
After exercise, insulin sensitivity can remain high for several hours. It is therefore important to monitor blood sugar levels, adjust carbohydrate intake and ensure adequate recovery.

Education and awareness :
Teammates, coaches and other team members should be informed about the athlete's diabetes, the signs of hypoglycaemia and what to do in an emergency.

Although managing diabetes in sportspeople requires adjustments and special attention, it should never be an obstacle to participation in sport. With proper planning, careful monitoring and the support of a medical team, diabetic athletes can excel in their sport and reap the full benefits of sport while effectively managing their condition.

Importance of hormones in sports performance.

Hormones play a central role in regulating many bodily functions, and their influence naturally extends to sports performance. From muscle growth and stress response to energy and recovery, hormones are key players that can help or hinder an athlete's ability to reach their maximum potential. Here's a fluid overview of the importance of hormones in sports performance.

The world of sport is an orchestrated dance of precision, endurance and strength, with every movement influenced by a complex network of hormones. Think adrenaline, which prepares the body for 'fight or flight' by increasing the heart rate, blood flow to the muscles and the release of energy. In the heat of competition, it's adrenaline that can push an athlete beyond his or her limits.

During training, it is testosterone, in both men and women, that plays a crucial role in muscle growth, strength and recovery. This anabolic hormone helps repair and grow the muscle fibres stressed during exercise. So it's not surprising that testosterone is at the heart of many discussions about doping in sport.

Growth hormone also has a role to play. It is involved in tissue regeneration, muscle growth and the response to the stress of intense exercise. Its influence does not stop with growth during childhood, and it remains a pillar of muscle recovery and development in adulthood.

However, performance is not just about growth and strength. Endurance is just as crucial, and here the stress hormone cortisol comes into play. Although often considered harmful because of its catabolic effects, cortisol, when released in response to exercise, helps to mobilise energy reserves and regulate metabolism.

At the same time, insulin plays an essential role in energy management, helping to regulate blood glucose and promote its absorption by the muscles, providing the fuel needed for physical activity.

Every athlete, whether consciously or not, dances to the rhythm of these hormones. But, like any dance, balance is essential. Hormonal imbalance, whether due to overtraining, stress or other external factors, can hamper an athlete's performance, recovery and overall health.

Understanding and respecting the role of hormones in sports performance is essential for optimising training, competition and recovery. In this hormonal symphony, every note counts, and it is harmony that leads to true athletic excellence.

Support of the endocrine athlete.

Supporting athletes suffering from endocrine disorders requires a multi-dimensional approach that takes into account medical specificities, sporting requirements and psychological needs. Each endocrine disorder presents its own challenges, but careful management can help athletes achieve their goals while maintaining their health.

1. In-depth medical assessment :
First and foremost, the athlete must undergo a full medical assessment to understand the nature and severity of his or her endocrine disorder. This assessment will provide a basis for drawing up a suitable treatment and training plan.

2. Individual training planning :
Athletes with endocrine disorders may require modifications to their training programme. For example, a diabetic athlete will have to adjust the intensity and duration of training according to their blood sugar levels.

3. Education and self-monitoring :
Athletes need to be well informed about their condition, the symptoms to watch out for and what to do if something

goes wrong. In the case of diabetes, this means training in how to monitor blood sugar levels, administer insulin and manage hypo- or hyperglycaemia.

4. Food and nutrition :
Work with a specialist dietician to develop a meal plan that supports both the athlete's energy needs and the management of their endocrine disorder.

5. Communication with the management team :
It is essential that coaches, physiotherapists and other members of the support team are informed of the athlete's condition, any limitations and the emergency measures to be taken.

6. Psychological support :
Managing an endocrine disorder can be emotionally challenging, especially in the competitive context of sport. Access to psychological support, whether in the form of therapy or support groups, can be beneficial.

7. Preparing for the competition :
Special measures may be required on competition days. For example, a diabetic athlete may need to check his blood sugar levels more frequently and adjust his carbohydrate intake and treatment accordingly.

8. Recovery and rest :
Certain endocrine disorders can affect an athlete's ability to recover. It is crucial to ensure adequate recovery to avoid any complications.

9. Interdisciplinary collaboration :
The endocrine athlete will benefit from a coordinated approach to care, involving endocrinologists, sports doctors, dieticians, psychologists and other relevant specialists.

Although the presence of an endocrine condition can present additional challenges for the athlete, with the right guidance, education and support, it is entirely possible to achieve sporting excellence while effectively managing the medical condition.

Prevention of disorders endocrinology related to sport.

Sport, while beneficial to overall health, can, in certain circumstances, contribute to endocrine disorders or exacerbate pre-existing conditions. Effective prevention requires an understanding of the associated risks and a proactive approach to minimising them.

1. Female athlete syndrome (FAS) :
This syndrome has three interrelated components: menstrual disorders, low bone density and eating disorders. To prevent FAS, you need to :
- Raising awareness of the dangers of eating disorders.
- Watch for signs of under-nutrition or over-training.
- Encourage a balanced diet.
- Make sure you get enough calcium and vitamin D for healthy bones.

2. Hypogonadism of hypothalamic origin (HH) in men :
Just as women can experience menstrual irregularities due to intense training, some male athletes can experience a drop in testosterone production due to physiological stress. Prevention includes:
- Recognise the signs, such as low libido, fatigue or loss of muscle mass.
- Ensure proper nutrition and rest.
- Balance the intensity and duration of training.

3. Disturbances in thyroid function :
Endurance athletes, in particular, may experience variations in thyroid function. To minimise the risk :
- Regular monitoring of thyroid hormone levels in elite athletes.
- Make sure you get enough iodine, which is essential for the production of thyroid hormones.

4. Hypoglycaemia in diabetic athletes :
Intense physical activity can lead to a rapid drop in blood sugar levels in diabetic athletes.
- Educate the athlete about adjusting insulin and carbohydrate intake before, during and after exercise.
- Encourage regular monitoring of blood sugar levels.

5. Osteoporosis :
Low bone density can be a concern, particularly in female athletes with irregular or absent periods.
- Make sure you get enough calcium and vitamin D.
- Encourage weight-bearing exercises to build bone density.

6. Education and awareness :
To provide athletes, coaches and medical teams with information on the potential risks of sport-related endocrine disorders.

7. Regular checks :
Regular medical check-ups, including blood tests, can help detect and manage endocrine disorders before they become a problem.

The key to preventing sport-related endocrinological disorders lies in a balanced approach to training, appropriate nutrition, ongoing education and careful medical monitoring. Open communication between athletes, coaches and health professionals is essential to ensure the athlete's well-being and optimum performance.

Chapter 13:
ENDOCRINOLOGY IN DIFFERENT CULTURES

Intercultural approach in endocrinology.

The cross-cultural approach to endocrinology recognises that cultural factors can have a significant impact on how patients perceive, understand and manage their endocrine conditions. Cultural differences can influence attitudes towards disease, beliefs about causes and treatments, and health-related behaviours. It is therefore essential for healthcare professionals to take these nuances into account in order to provide appropriate, respectful and effective care.

1. Perceptions of the disease :
In some cultures, endocrine diseases, such as diabetes or thyroid disorders, may be perceived as curses, the result of past actions or even divine punishments. Understanding these beliefs is crucial to approaching the patient with empathy and providing appropriate education.

2. Beliefs about treatment :
While the Western approach often favours drugs and medical interventions, other cultures may value traditional remedies, spiritual interventions or specific dietary approaches. Working with the patient to integrate these beliefs into a treatment plan can improve adherence and outcomes.

3. Communication and consent :
In some cultures, discussing a diagnosis or prognosis directly with the patient may be considered inappropriate. The family may play a central role in medical decision-making. Healthcare professionals must be sensitive to

these nuances and ensure that informed consent is obtained in accordance with the patient's cultural norms.

4. Diet and lifestyle :
Eating habits vary considerably from one culture to another. These differences can have a significant impact on endocrine diseases, particularly diabetes. Dietary recommendations need to be adapted according to cultural preferences and habits.

5. Gender issues :
Cultural gender norms can influence the management of endocrine disorders. For example, in some cultures, discussions about menstrual disorders or fertility may be taboo. Healthcare professionals must approach these subjects with sensitivity and discretion.

6. Education and resources :
Providing educational resources in the patient's mother tongue, adapted to their literacy level and incorporating relevant cultural elements, can improve understanding and adherence to treatment.

7. Intercultural training for professionals :
It is essential that healthcare professionals receive specific training to understand and navigate intercultural complexities. This will not only improve the quality of care, but also strengthen trust and collaboration between patient and professional.
An intercultural approach to endocrinology requires recognition of and respect for cultural differences. By adopting an attitude of listening, learning and adapting, healthcare professionals can offer personalised care that meets the unique needs of each patient.

Managing beliefs and traditional practices.

Managing traditional beliefs and practices in medical care, particularly in endocrinology, is a complex challenge. Traditional beliefs can profoundly influence how a patient perceives their illness, its causes, treatment and prognosis. For healthcare professionals, it is essential to navigate this landscape sensitively, respectfully and effectively.

1. Listening and understanding :
The first step is to listen actively to the patient. Try to understand their beliefs, concerns and any traditional practices they may follow. Asking open, non-judgmental questions creates a safe environment for dialogue.

2. Education and information :
Once you understand the patient's perspective, present clear, factual medical information about the condition, treatment options and expected outcomes. It is essential to adapt this education to the patient's level of literacy and cultural understanding.

3. Integrating traditional practices :
Where possible and safe, consider incorporating some of the traditional practices or remedies into the treatment plan. For example, certain traditional herbs or techniques may be beneficial when used in conjunction with conventional treatments.

4. Dealing with conflict :
If there is a conflict between traditional practices and medical recommendations, it is crucial to approach the subject with empathy. Clearly explain the reasons for your recommendations and the potential risks associated with traditional practices. Look for common ground or

alternatives that respect the patient's beliefs while guaranteeing their safety.

5. Working with traditional healers :
In some communities, working with traditional healers can be beneficial. These healers are often highly trusted within their communities and can play an essential role in guiding health beliefs and practices.

6. Community support :
Engaging with the wider community, by organising education sessions or workshops, can help to break down barriers and build mutual understanding. It can also help to demystify certain preconceived ideas and promote safer health practices.

7. Further training :
It is essential for healthcare professionals to regularly learn about the cultural practices and beliefs of the populations they serve. Intercultural training can provide tools and strategies to navigate these complexities effectively.

8. Interprofessional networking :
Collaborate with other healthcare professionals who have expertise or experience in cross-cultural care. This can provide additional support, resources and strategies for managing challenges.

Managing traditional beliefs and practices in endocrinology requires a respectful, patient-centred and collaborative approach. By recognising and valuing the unique perspectives and experiences of each patient, healthcare professionals can provide truly holistic and personalised care.

Raising awareness of the specific needs of different populations.

Awareness of the specific health needs of different populations is crucial to providing equitable and effective care. Each population, whether defined by ethnicity, religion, gender, age, sexual orientation or any other factor, has its own challenges, beliefs and practices that can influence the way they perceive and manage their health. Here's a fluid approach to raising awareness:

In the vast world of medicine, each individual carries with them a mosaic of cultures, experiences and identities. Each piece of this mosaic reflects not only his or her personal history, but also the shared histories, beliefs and expectations of his or her community. When we talk about raising awareness of the specific needs of different populations, it is not just a question of understanding this mosaic, but also of recognising how it influences the individual's care pathway.

Take, for example, an older woman from an ethnic minority, who may face language barriers, cultural beliefs about illness and stigma attached to her age or gender. For her, navigating the healthcare system could be a completely different experience to that of a young man living in an urban environment with easy access to health information and services.

Awareness begins with the recognition that each individual is unique, but also that they are the product of a complexity of interacting factors that influence their health. This implies ongoing training for healthcare professionals, who need to keep abreast of the issues specific to the different populations they serve. This training can address issues such as health disparities, intercultural communication, traditional health beliefs and systemic barriers to access to care.

But beyond training, it is essential to adopt an attitude of active listening and empathy. Ask open-ended questions, be curious and, above all, be respectful of the answers. Recognise that sometimes a patient's beliefs or practices may differ from your own, but that they are just as valid and important to them.

Finally, don't forget that awareness also means action. This means advocating policies that reduce health inequalities, working with communities to understand and respond to their needs, and always seeking to improve access, quality and appropriateness of care for every individual.

By integrating these principles into their practice, healthcare professionals can ensure that they meet not only the medical needs of their patients, but also their human, cultural and social needs, thereby providing truly patient-centred care.

Adapting care
depending on the cultural context.

Adapting medical care to the cultural context is essential if patients are to be treated comprehensively and with respect. Medicine is essentially a science, but the way it is perceived and practised is greatly influenced by culture. So if we are to offer relevant and empathetic care, it is essential to integrate this cultural dimension. Here is an integrated approach to this adaptation:

When a doctor places his stethoscope on a patient's chest, he is listening to more than just the heartbeat; he is connecting with the patient's history, beliefs and values.

This simple gesture becomes a bridge between medical science and the patient's cultural universe.

1. Knowledge and awareness :
It is essential for healthcare professionals to become familiar with the diverse cultures they are likely to encounter in their practice. This may involve understanding beliefs about illness, death and family, as well as dietary or religious practices that may influence care.

2. Effective communication :
This may mean using interpreters where language barriers exist, but it also means understanding non-verbal communication, which can vary from one culture to another. The way questions are asked, the level of eye contact and even physical proximity during interaction can all have cultural meanings.

3. Respect for beliefs and practices :
It is crucial to approach each patient with an open mind, without judgement. If a patient follows a traditional practice or has a particular belief about their illness, the professional should work with them to integrate these beliefs into the treatment plan if possible.

4. Shared decision-making :
In some cultural contexts, medical decisions are not taken solely by the patient, but in collaboration with the family or community. It is crucial to recognise these dynamics and integrate them into the care process.

5. Adapted education :
Provide medical information in a way that is culturally relevant and accessible. This may involve visual aids, brochures in different languages, or even community workshops.

6. Working with traditional healers :
In many cultures, healers play an essential role in health and well-being. Working with them can build trust and improve patient outcomes.

7. Flexibility :
Adapting care to a cultural context also means being flexible. This may mean modifying treatment plans, appointment times or even medical protocols to meet a patient's cultural needs.

Adapting medical care to the cultural context is not a luxury, but a necessity. In a globalised world, where borders are increasingly blurred, medical care must transcend cultural boundaries to touch the very essence of humanity: the desire for health, well-being and mutual respect.

Chapter 14:
PHARMACOLOGY IN ENDOCRINOLOGY

Commonly used medicines and their mechanism of action.

In the field of endocrinology, a large number of drugs are used to treat various disorders. These drugs act in different ways to modulate or replace endogenous hormones. Here is a list of drugs commonly used in endocrinology, together with their mechanism of action:

1. Insulin (used in the treatment of diabetes) :

Mechanism of action: Insulin regulates the concentration of glucose in the blood by promoting its entry into cells, particularly muscle and fat cells. It also inhibits glucose production by the liver.

2. Metformin (treatment of type 2 diabetes) :

Mechanism of action: Metformin reduces hepatic glucose production and improves insulin sensitivity, thereby improving peripheral glucose utilisation.

3. Levothyroxine (treatment of hypothyroidism) :

Mechanism of action: It is a synthetic form of T4 thyroid hormone. It replaces or supplements endogenous thyroid hormones, thereby improving the symptoms of hypothyroidism.

4. Antithyroid drugs (such as propylthiouracil and methimazole) :

Mechanism of action: They inhibit the synthesis of thyroid hormones by the thyroid gland, used to treat hyperthyroidism.

5. Corticosteroids (such as prednisone, used in a variety of conditions) :

Mechanism of action: These drugs are synthetic analogues of hormones produced by the adrenal glands. They have anti-inflammatory and immunosuppressive effects and influence the metabolism of carbohydrates, proteins and fats.

6. Aromatase inhibitors (such as anastrozole, used in certain breast cancers):

Mechanism of action: These drugs inhibit the enzyme aromatase, which converts androgens into oestrogens. By reducing oestrogen levels, they can help treat certain hormone-dependent breast cancers.

7. Bisphosphonates (such as alendronate, used in osteoporosis) :

Mechanism of action: These drugs inhibit bone resorption, thereby reducing bone loss and increasing bone mineral density.

8. GnRH agonists (such as leuprolide, used in endometriosis, fibroids and certain cancers):

Mechanism of action: These drugs modulate the release of gonadotropic hormones (LH and FSH) by the pituitary gland, thereby affecting the production of sex hormones such as oestrogen and testosterone.

This is only a partial list of the drugs used in endocrinology, but it gives an idea of the diversity of the mechanisms of action of these therapeutic agents. It is always advisable to consult a specialist for specific information about a drug or treatment.

Drug interactions to watch out for.

Drug interactions can alter the efficacy of medicines or increase the risk of side effects. In endocrinology, given the delicate nature of hormonal balance, it is particularly crucial to be aware of these interactions. Here are some of the common drug interactions to watch out for in this area:

1. Levothyroxine :
   - **Calcium and iron supplements**: These may reduce the absorption of levothyroxine. It is generally recommended that these supplements be taken several hours apart from levothyroxine.
   - **Antacids** containing aluminium or magnesium: May reduce the absorption of levothyroxine.
2. Insulin and hypoglycaemic drugs :
   - **Beta-blockers**: They can mask the symptoms of hypoglycaemia and reduce the hypoglycaemic response.
   - **Thiazides**: May increase blood sugar levels, requiring adjustment of insulin dose.
3. Antithyroid drugs (e.g. propylthiouracil) :
   - **Anticoagulants**: The anticoagulant effect may be increased, increasing the risk of bleeding.
   - **Beta-blockers**: Increased risk of side effects such as bradycardia.
4. Corticosteroids :
   - **Non-steroidal anti-inflammatory drugs (NSAIDs)**: Increases the risk of gastrointestinal ulcers and bleeding.
   - **Diuretics**: Increased risk of electrolyte imbalance, particularly hypokalaemia.
5. GnRH agonists :
   - **Oestrogens and progestins**: May reduce the efficacy of GnRH agonists.
6. Bisphosphonates :
   - **Antacids**: May interfere with the absorption of bisphosphonates.
   - **Aspirin**: Increases the risk of gastric irritation.
7. Medications for type 2 diabetes (such as metformin) :
   - **Iodine contrasts** used for imaging: May increase the risk of lactic acidosis in patients taking metformin.
8. Aromatase inhibitors :
   - **Drugs containing estrogens**: May reduce the efficacy of aromatase inhibitors.

It is crucial to note that this list is far from exhaustive. Patients should always inform their doctor of all the medicines, supplements and herbal remedies they are taking. In addition, regular consultation of a reliable pharmacological database or specialist pharmacist is essential for healthcare professionals to minimise the risk of harmful drug interactions.

The importance of adherence to treatment.

Adherence to treatment, i.e. the degree to which a patient follows medical recommendations regarding medication, diet or other lifestyle modifications, is a fundamental element of therapeutic success. Good adherence optimises treatment efficacy, improves patient outcomes and reduces healthcare costs. Here is a fluid discussion of its importance:

Imagine a gardener sowing seeds in a field, hoping for a bountiful harvest. He knows that for these seeds to germinate and produce, he must water them regularly, protect them from pests and provide them with the appropriate nutrients. If, for any reason, he neglects this care, the harvest is likely to be poor. In the same way, medical treatment can be seen as a seed that the doctor plants to improve the patient's health. However, without the patient's proper support, this seed may not produce the desired results.

Optimising treatment effectiveness: Just as a plant needs regular watering to grow, a treatment needs to be taken regularly to work properly. For example, omitting doses of antibiotics can not only reduce their effectiveness, but also contribute to drug resistance.

Preventing complications: If a plant is left unattended, it can be invaded by parasites or diseases. Similarly, if a patient does not follow their treatment regime, they may be exposed to complications. In diabetes, for example, poor adherence can lead to serious complications such as blindness, neuropathy or heart problems.

Saving health resources: A far-sighted gardener who looks after his garden from the outset avoids the cost and effort of dealing with problems later. Similarly, good adherence can reduce the need for hospital admissions, costly treatments and other medical interventions.

Empowering the patient: A gardener who sees his plants flourish thanks to his efforts feels valued and confident. A patient who adheres to his treatment and sees improvements in his health also feels autonomous and in control of his life.

Strengthening the doctor-patient relationship: Just as a gardener might seek advice from experts or other gardeners, a patient needs to trust his or her doctor to follow his or her recommendations. Good adherence strengthens this relationship of trust and paves the way for more open communication.

As with a garden, the success of treatment depends as much on the day-to-day care as on the quality of the seeds. Raising awareness of the importance of adherence and providing the tools to support this adherence are essential to ensure that every patient has the best chance of living a healthy life.

Common side effects
and their management.

Endocrine medicines, like all medicines, can have side effects. Knowledge of these side effects and how to manage them is crucial for both the healthcare professional and the patient. Let's tackle this subject by talking about the common side effects of certain endocrine medicines and their management strategies, keeping to a fluid and integrated style.

In the journey that is medical treatment, side effects can be compared to unexpected bumps in the road. They can occur at any time, but with proper preparation and response, they can often be managed or mitigated.

Take, for example, **levothyroxine**, used to treat hypothyroidism. If the dose is too high, the patient may experience symptoms of hyperthyroidism, such as palpitations, agitation or insomnia. In this case, the route to successful treatment may require a revision of the dose. Regular monitoring of TSH (thyroid-stimulating hormone) levels and symptoms enables treatment to be fine-tuned.

Speaking of **diabetes**, hypoglycaemic drugs such as insulin can sometimes lead to hypoglycaemia, a situation comparable to a sudden and unexpected bend in the road. Immediate management would involve eating fast carbohydrates, such as sweetened juice or sweets. To avoid future episodes, it would be essential to review diet and exercise, and possibly adjust the dose of medication.

Corticosteroids, powerful anti-inflammatory drugs, may seem like a high-speed motorway for treating inflammation and autoimmune reactions. However, this road has its tolls in the form of side effects such as weight gain, osteoporosis and insomnia. To manage these effects, it is often recommended to take the drug in the morning, adopt a diet rich in calcium and vitamin D, and regularly monitor bone density.

Finally, osteoporosis drugs such as **bisphosphonates** have their own set of obstacles. They can cause gastrointestinal problems or, rarely, osteonecrosis of the jaw. One strategy for avoiding these problems could be to take the drug on an empty stomach, stand for 30 minutes after taking it, and practise good dental hygiene.
The key to this therapeutic journey is open communication between patient and healthcare professional. Knowing the route, anticipating the bends and having a plan for each obstacle means that the journey can continue safely and reach the desired destination: better health.

Chapter 15:
HOLISTIC APPROACH
IN ENDOCRINOLOGY

The importance of balance between body, mind and soul.

Harmony between body, mind and soul is often seen as an ideal of complete well-being. This interconnected trinity shapes our experience of life, our response to challenges and our search for meaning. Let's plunge together into a fluid reflection on the importance of this balance.

Imagine a musical instrument, such as a violin. The body of the instrument, made of carved wood, could be compared to our physical body, offering structure and form. The melodies it produces evoke our mind, with its thoughts, emotions and consciousness. The passion and intention behind each note played embody the soul, that intangible spark that gives depth and meaning to our existence.

The body: Like the violin, our body needs maintenance. It needs proper nutrition, exercise and rest to function optimally. When it is well maintained, it becomes a precise and responsive instrument, capable of transforming our intentions into actions and our thoughts into reality.

Mind: Melodies played on the violin can evoke a variety of emotions, just as our minds navigate through a range of thoughts and feelings every day. Mental health is as important as physical health. A healthy mind allows us to interpret the world around us, make thoughtful decisions and build meaningful relationships.

The soul: This is the energy that drives the violinist, the passion that brings the music to life. Similarly, our soul is that inner part that seeks meaning, yearns for connection and guides our moral compass. It nourishes our sense of identity, our desire to belong and our quest for a greater purpose.

When these three elements are in harmony, the individual feels complete, balanced and aligned. However, just as a violin can go out of tune, imbalances can arise between our body, mind and soul. Ignoring any one of these aspects can lead to feelings of unease, frustration or emptiness.

Recognising the importance of this balance is the first step towards holistic well-being. This involves listening to your body's needs, nourishing your mind with positive thoughts and connecting with your soul through spiritual practices, meditation or creativity.

In the medical field, the importance of this balance is increasingly recognised. Holistic approaches, which integrate care for body, mind and soul, offer a more complete perspective on health and well-being.
So, like the violinist who, with passion and practice, seeks to master each note, each of us is invited to seek this balance, to refine our inner harmony, and to play the unique and precious melody of our lives.

Complementary techniques: meditation, yoga, acupuncture.

The constant evolution of modern medicine has highlighted the importance of complementary and alternative therapies. Among these, meditation, yoga and acupuncture have gained particular recognition for their ability to promote overall well-being. Let's integrate these three practices into a fluid and coherent exploration of their benefits.

Think of health and well-being as a vast landscape. At the heart of this landscape is a serene river, symbolising our inner balance. This river is fed by three essential tributaries: meditation, yoga and acupuncture.

1. Meditation :

It's like a spring of pure water flowing into our inner river. By devoting oneself to meditation, the individual refocuses, finding a moment of peace in the daily hustle and bustle. Meditation helps to clear the mind, manage stress and strengthen self-awareness. Regular practice can reduce anxiety, improve concentration and cultivate a deep sense of inner peace.

2. Yoga :

It can be compared to a vitalising current, stimulating the flow of the river. It is an ancient practice that unites body and mind through a series of postures, breathing techniques and meditations. Yoga strengthens the body, improves flexibility and promotes deep relaxation. By harmonising breath with movement, yoga invites conscious presence, strengthening the link between the physical and the mental.

3. Acupuncture :

Think of this practice as a tributary that corrects the course of the river, unblocking obstacles and restoring the natural flow. Based on traditional Chinese medicine, acupuncture involves inserting fine needles into specific points on the body. These points are considered energy centres, and stimulating them aims to rebalance the flow of energy, or 'Qi', in the body. Acupuncture is known to relieve pain, reduce stress and treat a range of conditions, from digestive disorders to migraines.

Just as the three tributaries nourish and enrich the river, meditation, yoga and acupuncture complement each other, offering a holistic approach to well-being. By incorporating these techniques into our routine, we can not only treat specific ailments, but also build resilience, improve emotional balance and cultivate a deep connection with our inner selves.

In a world often marked by stress and haste, these practices remind us of the importance of pausing, listening and looking after ourselves, guiding individuals towards deeper harmony with themselves and the world around them.

The importance of a patient-centred.

At the heart of modern medicine lies a crucial transformation: the shift from disease-centred medicine to patient-centred medicine. This individualised approach recognises each patient as a unique entity, with his or her own experiences, values and needs. Let's look together, in fluid style, at the importance of this patient-centred approach.

Imagine an art studio where every canvas is treated in the same way, regardless of subject, colour or style. Although each work would receive the same attention, the result would not do justice to the uniqueness of each creation. In the same way, to treat each patient according to a single model without considering their individuality is to neglect the unique picture of their life.

Holistic understanding: A patient-centred approach seeks to understand the whole picture - not just the clinical symptoms, but also the patient's emotions, beliefs, history and aspirations. It's like recognising every nuance and detail of a work of art.

Therapeutic partnership: Instead of seeing the doctor-patient relationship as a simple transmission of information, it becomes a genuine partnership. Like two artists working together on a canvas, doctor and patient work hand in hand to co-create the best path to health.

Patient autonomy: Valuing the patient's expertise in his or her own life is essential. It's like giving artists the power to choose their colours and techniques. Incorporating the patient's preferences and values into the treatment plan encourages greater adherence and satisfaction.

Effective communication: Attentive listening and open communication are at the heart of this approach. Just as an art critic seeks to understand the artist's vision, the doctor strives to understand the patient's perspective.

Emotional support: Recognising and responding to patients' emotional needs is as important as treating their physical symptoms. It's like caring for the soul of a work of art, not just its surface.

Shared decision-making: In this collaboration, the doctor offers his medical expertise while the patient contributes his intimate knowledge of his own body and life. Together, they make informed, mutually agreed decisions.

By putting the patient at the centre, medicine recognises that behind every diagnosis lies a story, a personality and a unique set of experiences. It is an invitation to see beyond the symptoms, to listen with empathy and to embrace the delicate and profoundly human art of healing. Ultimately, a patient-centred approach makes medicine not just a science, but an art.

Working with alternative or complementary professionals.

Health and well-being are like a vast orchestra in which each instrument, although distinct, contributes to the overall symphony. In the same way, the collaboration between traditional health professionals and those of alternative or complementary therapies creates a holistic melody of care. Explore this complex harmony and how it enriches the medical landscape.

At the heart of a concert hall, imagine the traditional doctor as the first violin, playing the main melody, based on centuries of medical research and clinical expertise. But around him, there are other instruments, representing alternative or complementary therapists, each bringing a nuance, a depth, and sometimes even a totally new perspective to the composition.

1. Naturopaths: They can be compared to flutes, bringing a natural sweetness to the whole. They focus on natural healing, prevention and balance, using remedies such as medicinal plants, nutrition and other traditional therapies.

2. Chiropractors: Think of them as double basses, providing structure and support. Their expertise focuses on the spine and musculoskeletal system, helping to align the body and improve nerve function.

3. Acupuncturists: They are like harps, touching delicate points to evoke profound responses. Based on traditional Chinese medicine, acupuncture aims to balance the body's vital energy, or "Qi", by stimulating specific points.

4. Massage therapists: Like percussion, they use touch to relieve tension and promote relaxation. Massages can improve circulation, reduce stress and relieve muscle pain.

5. Meditation and yoga practitioners: Think of them as the wooden winds, bringing calm and concentration to the whole. They promote self-awareness, mental balance and bodily flexibility.

When these professionals work together, in harmony with the primary physician, the symphony of care is rich and nuanced. Each therapist brings his or her own expertise, but it is their collaboration that enables an integrated approach to well-being.

The doctor, as coordinator, needs to be informed of the complementary therapies the patient is receiving to ensure that they complement each other and do not conflict. Patients, for their part, need to feel confident in sharing their therapeutic choices and seeking balanced advice.

The beauty of this collaboration is that, while respecting the fundamental principles of evidence-based medicine, it recognises and integrates the virtues of traditional, alternative and complementary therapies, offering a wider range of therapeutic options.

Chapter 16:
GLOBAL HEALTH ISSUES
IN ENDOCRINOLOGY

Epidemiology of endocrine disorders worldwide.

Epidemiology, the science that studies the distribution, determinants and dynamics of disease in populations, offers a valuable window into the prevalence and incidence of endocrine disorders around the world. Let's embark on a journey through this global medical landscape, exploring how hormonal imbalances affect different regions and cultures.

Imagine the Earth seen from space, a luminous globe with areas of intense light and others more subdued. These points of light could symbolise the regions where certain endocrine disorders are predominant, offering a global view of the challenges and trends in endocrine health.

1. Diabetes :
One of the most widespread endocrine disorders, diabetes, is particularly prevalent in many parts of the world. In North America and parts of the Middle East, the prevalence of type 2 diabetes is particularly high, largely due to a sedentary lifestyle, a high-calorie diet and other lifestyle factors. In addition, developing nations, with rapid changes in lifestyle and diet, are also seeing an alarming increase in cases.

2. Thyroid disorders :
Europe, particularly Central Europe, has historically been an endemic area for iodine deficiency, an essential element for thyroid function. Although the situation has improved

with universal salt iodisation, cases of goitre and other thyroid disorders persist. In Asia, certain regions also have high rates of thyroid disease, including thyroid cancer.

3. Reproductive disorders :

In various parts of Africa and Asia, there is a high prevalence of reproductive disorders such as polycystic ovary syndrome (PCOS) and infertility. Genetic, environmental and cultural factors all play a role in this epidemiology.

4. Osteoporosis :

Regions with limited exposure to sunlight, such as Northern Europe, have a higher prevalence of osteoporosis, partly due to a lack of vitamin D, which is essential for bone health.

5. Endocrine cancers :

Some geographical areas, notably East Asia, have higher rates of specific cancers, such as thyroid cancer. The reasons for these variations are not always clear, but they could involve genetic, environmental and dietary factors.

Returning to our view from space, it is crucial to recognise that these bright spots of incidence and prevalence are not static. Over time, lifestyles, the environment, access to healthcare and awareness influence the dynamics of these endocrine disorders. However, thanks to epidemiology, researchers and healthcare professionals can better understand, prevent and treat these conditions, working tirelessly to make the overall picture of endocrine health brighter for everyone.

Challenges and opportunities
in countries with limited resources.

In countries with limited resources, endocrine medicine, like other medical specialities, presents itself as a complex jigsaw puzzle of challenges interwoven with unexpected opportunities. It's like a winding road through rugged terrain, where every difficult bend reveals a panorama of renewed possibilities and hopes.

The first major difficulty in these regions is limited access to healthcare. Faced with alarming symptoms, many people do not have the means or the geographical proximity to consult a specialist, leaving endocrine disorders undiagnosed or poorly treated. But in this shadow, an opportunity is emerging: that of telemedicine. Thanks to advances in technology, even a basic smartphone can serve as a bridge between an isolated patient and a specialist, offering invaluable medical diagnosis or advice.

Secondly, the lack of specialised equipment and medicines makes it difficult to treat patients. Without the right tools, diagnosis and treatment of endocrine disorders can be hampered. However, this constraint has stimulated frugal innovation and the adaptation of existing tools to meet local needs. For example, the use of simplified diagnostic tools or the training of community health workers to administer basic care.

Awareness and education are also major challenges. Myths, stigma and lack of information can lead to delays in diagnosis or inappropriate treatment. But here again, there is an opportunity: community education campaigns, school programmes or local health ambassadors can enlighten communities about endocrine disorders and encourage timely care.

Limited financial resources often make it difficult to purchase medicines or pay for consultations. However, this has prompted many countries to explore innovative financing models, such as micro-insurance or public-private partnerships, to make healthcare accessible to all.

Finally, specialist training can be scarce, with few endocrinologists available for a large population. Yet hidden within this challenge is the opportunity for distance learning programmes, twinning with international institutions or intensive courses to equip general practitioners with basic endocrine skills.

Navigating this winding road, countries with limited resources illustrate an essential lesson: resilience in the face of adversity. With each challenge encountered, creativity, collaboration and determination spring to life, shaping a future where, despite the obstacles, endocrine health becomes accessible to everyone, everywhere.

International collaboration and exchange programmes.

International collaboration and exchange programmes in the medical field are like bridges built between different nations and cultures, opening up avenues for the sharing of knowledge, skills and resources. Think of this collaboration as a great web woven of interconnected threads, each thread representing a nation, an institution or an individual, working together to create a global image of progress and innovation.

At the heart of this web, exchange programmes are the shuttles that weave these threads together. They enable healthcare professionals, whether students, researchers or clinicians, to travel from one region to another, immerse themselves in a new medical culture, and bring home fresh perspectives and enriched skills.

One of the most obvious benefits of these exchanges is the transfer of knowledge. An endocrinologist from a developed country, for example, can share recent advances in the diagnosis or treatment of endocrine disorders with his or her counterparts in a developing country. Conversely, the same endocrinologist could learn about traditional approaches or innovative methods of disease management adapted to limited resources.

But beyond sharing knowledge, these exchanges also cultivate a deep cultural understanding. Each healthcare system reflects the values, beliefs and traditions of its society. By immersing themselves in a different medical environment, healthcare professionals acquire the cultural sensitivity that is essential for truly patient-centred medicine in a globalised world.

These programmes also stimulate collaborative research. Faced with global medical challenges such as the COVID-19 pandemic and the rise of diabetes, international collaboration is essential to unite efforts, share data and accelerate discoveries.
International collaboration also builds capacity. Through institutional partnerships, hospitals and universities can benefit from equipment, training or resources, thereby improving the quality and efficiency of their care.

Finally, for professionals at the start of their careers, these exchanges offer an invaluable opportunity to network, establish contacts with mentors or colleagues abroad, and lay the foundations for future collaborations.
Take another look at this web, where each woven thread strengthens the overall picture. International collaborations and exchange programmes, with their multifaceted interactions, enrich the medical landscape, building a

global community where mutual support, innovation and understanding lead to better health for all.

Endocrinology in the face of global crises: pandemics, climate change.

Faced with the growing scale of global crises such as pandemics and climate change, endocrinology, like other medical fields, finds itself at a crossroads of adaptation, innovation and reflection. Imagine this medical speciality as a lighthouse in the midst of a storm, seeking to guide endocrine patients through turbulent waters, while adapting its beam to new challenges.

Pandemics :
The sudden appearance of global infectious diseases, such as COVID-19, has direct and indirect ramifications for endocrinology. Directly, it has been observed that patients with endocrine disorders, particularly diabetes, may be more vulnerable to severe forms of these diseases. This has led to an in-depth examination of how hormonal imbalances can interact with infectious agents and affect the outcome of disease. Indirectly, confinements and disruptions to the healthcare system have posed challenges for the ongoing management of endocrine disorders, from regular monitoring to surgical interventions.

Climate change :
These global upheavals have a multitude of effects on health, including endocrine function. Rising temperatures, for example, can affect temperature regulation in patients suffering from certain endocrine disorders. More broadly, extreme weather events can disrupt the production and distribution of essential medicines such as insulin. In addition, environmental contamination resulting from

climate change can introduce endocrine disruptors into the food chain, affecting the hormonal function of individuals.

But beyond the challenges, these crises also offer a unique opportunity for reinvention. In response to the pandemic, endocrinology has embraced telemedicine, offering remote consultations, virtual follow-ups and online therapeutic education. This has not only ensured continuity of care in times of crisis, but has also paved the way for more flexible and accessible models of care in the future.

Climate change, meanwhile, has been a catalyst for thinking about sustainability in medicine. Greener practices in endocrine laboratories, reduced use of plastics in medical devices, and greater awareness of endocrine disruptors are all steps towards a more environmentally-friendly endocrinology.

Navigating these tumultuous waters, endocrinology, armed with science, innovation and resilience, continues to light the way for its patients, while forging its own path to meet the challenges of an ever-changing world.

Chapter 17:
DIGITAL HEALTH AND ENDOCRINOLOGY

Mobile applications for monitoring and patient education.

In the digital age, mobile apps have revolutionised the way patients manage their health conditions and educate themselves about their illnesses. Think of these apps as personal assistants that are always at hand, offering advice, reminders and information in real time. In the field of endocrinology, these technological tools have added considerable value, transforming the patient-carer relationship and facilitating the self-management of endocrine conditions.

- Parameter monitoring :
  - Dedicated apps allow diabetic patients to track their blood sugar levels, record their insulin or medication intake, and monitor their diet and physical activity. Similarly, for those managing thyroid conditions, apps can help record symptoms, medication dosages and test results.
- Medication reminders :
  - Adherence to treatment is crucial in the management of endocrine disorders. Specially designed applications can send reminders to patients to take their medication on time, ensuring optimal therapeutic efficacy.

- Education and information :
  - Access to reliable information is a cornerstone of self-management. Applications can offer educational modules, videos, articles and other

resources to help patients better understand their condition and best management practices.
* Connectivity with healthcare professionals :

Some applications offer telemedicine features, enabling patients to consult their endocrinologist or a medical team via chat, call or video. This facilitates access to care, particularly for those living in remote areas.
* Communities and support :

Applications can also offer forums or discussion groups where patients can share their experiences, ask questions and find support from others in similar situations.
* Integration with other systems :

With the evolution of wearable technology, such as smartwatches or continuous glucose monitors, applications can synchronise with these devices to collect data in real time, offering a complete and instantaneous view of the patient's state of health.
* Educational   games for children :

For young patients, particularly those with type 1 diabetes, edutainment applications have been developed to teach self-management of the disease through games and interactive activities.

As the medical world continues to evolve towards a more patient-centred approach, mobile applications are positioning themselves as powerful tools for empowering individuals to manage their health. They embody the intersection of technology and care, promising a future where information, support and disease management are literally at your fingertips.

Use of connected objects (wearables) for real-time monitoring.

At the dawn of a new era in medicine, connected objects, often referred to as 'wearables', embody the fusion of technology and healthcare, transforming the medical landscape into a dynamic real-time monitoring picture. Imagine wearing a wristband or other gadget that not only tells the time or counts your steps, but also monitors vital parameters, detecting abnormalities before you even feel the slightest symptom. This is the promise of wearables in endocrinology and beyond.

1. Glucose monitoring :
One of the most revolutionary examples in endocrinology is the continuous glucose monitor (CGM). These devices, worn on the surface of the skin, measure glucose levels in the interstitial fluid in real time. For diabetics, this means the possibility of monitoring their levels without frequent blood sampling, while receiving alerts for impending hyperglycaemia or hypoglycaemia.

2. Insulin therapy management :
In conjunction with GCMs, insulin pumps can be adjusted in real time according to glucose readings, enabling more precise and personalised insulin delivery.

3. Monitoring physical activity :
Connected watches and fitness wristbands track physical activity, heart rate, sleep quality and other parameters. This data can help patients with endocrine disorders to adjust their disease management, particularly with regard to **the impact of exercise on metabolism.**

4. Weight loss support :
For patients with metabolic or endocrine disorders associated with obesity, wearables can track calorie intake, exercise and even sleep patterns, providing a holistic view of the factors influencing weight gain.

5. Stress monitoring :
Some devices can measure physiological markers of stress, such as heart rate variability. This is particularly useful for patients whose hormonal imbalances may be exacerbated by chronic stress.

6. Reminders and notifications :
Integrated with health applications, wearables can remind patients to take their medication, check their hormone levels or perform other tasks essential to managing their **condition.**

7. Data storage and sharing :
Connected objects can store data over the long term, enabling patients and healthcare professionals to examine trends, identify triggers or modify treatment accordingly.

While the promise of wearables is undeniable, it is also essential to navigate with caution, ensuring data security, device accuracy and the potential for information overload. Nevertheless, in a world where technology and health are becoming increasingly intertwined, connected objects are charting a course towards a future where the management of endocrine disorders is proactive, personalised and fully informed.

The platforms patient data management.

In today's medical landscape, data plays an essential role, serving as the foundation for high-quality, accurate and patient-centred healthcare. Patient data management platforms are like vast digital libraries, housing volumes of clinical information, offering healthcare professionals instant and integrated access to a patient's medical history. In this exploration, we dive into the world of data management platforms and discover how they are shaping the future of medicine.

1. Electronic medical records (EMR) :
At the heart of any data management platform is the EMR. This is a complete digital record of a patient's medical history, medications, allergies, laboratory results, X-ray images and much more. EMRs not only make it easier to store and access data, they also enable care to be coordinated between different specialists or institutions.

2. Patient portals :
These online platforms give patients direct access to their medical information, enabling them to consult their results, book appointments, renew prescriptions or communicate directly with their medical team.

3. Data analysis platforms :
As well as simply storing data, some platforms use advanced algorithms to analyse and interpret the information, identifying trends, anomalies or even predicting risks for the patient, helping healthcare professionals to make informed decisions.

4. Inter-system integration :
To ensure continuity of care, many platforms enable integration between different systems or institutions, ensuring that a patient's data is accessible whether they are seen in a local clinic or a major teaching hospital.

5. Security and confidentiality :
With cyber-attacks and privacy concerns on the rise, data management platforms are focusing on security, using advanced encryption protocols, two-factor authentication and other measures to protect sensitive information.

6. Interoperability :
In a world of rapidly evolving technology, interoperability - the ability of systems to communicate with each other - is essential. Modern platforms are designed to be compatible with a variety of tools, applications and devices, from a patient's glucose monitor to state-of-the-art imaging.

7. Artificial intelligence and machine learning :
Some platforms incorporate artificial intelligence (AI) to analyse the data, offering potential diagnoses, treatment

suggestions or even identifying patients at risk of certain complications.

As the volume of medical information grows exponentially, patient data management platforms are positioning themselves as the guardians of this precious resource. They are transforming mountains of data into actionable information, guiding clinical decisions and shaping an era of medicine where every decision is underpinned by a complete and integrated understanding of each patient's unique story.

The importance of cyber security in health.

In an interconnected world, where technology is deeply integrated into almost every aspect of our daily lives, cyber security in healthcare has become a crucial concern. Imagine a hospital as a fortress, protecting not only its patients physically, but also their precious digital data. However, as medicine advances and adopts new technologies, it also opens doors to potential vulnerabilities.

1. Protection of sensitive data :
Medical records contain a wealth of sensitive information, ranging from medical history to financial data. A security breach can put this data at risk, with devastating consequences for patients. Incidents of identity theft, fraud or extortion can result from a single data breach.

2. Integrity of medical systems :
In addition to the records themselves, many hospitals and clinics are equipped with connected medical devices. A breach in the security of these devices could disrupt their

operation or even render them inoperative, putting patients' lives at risk.

3. Continuity of care :
Cyber attacks, such as ransomware, can cripple a healthcare facility's systems, delaying or interrupting critical care, scheduled surgery or access to essential medicines.

4. Confidentiality :
Respect for privacy is a fundamental right of patients. A breach in cybersecurity could expose intimate details of a patient's life, creating embarrassing and even traumatic situations.

5. Regulatory compliance :
Many countries have introduced strict regulations concerning the protection of healthcare data. Violations of these regulations can result in severe penalties, substantial fines and a loss of trust on the part of patients and the public.

6. Research and development :
Medical data is essential for research and development. A breach could compromise ongoing studies, slow down the development of new treatments or drugs, and jeopardise research collaborations.

The importance of cyber security in healthcare is therefore undeniable. For every technological advance, it is essential to have a corresponding security strategy. This requires investment in secure infrastructures, regular staff training and constant monitoring of emerging threats.

As healthcare embraces the digital age, cybersecurity should be seen not as an afterthought, but as an intrinsic component of modern medicine. It is the shield that protects data integrity, confidentiality and availability, ensuring that medical technology remains a healing tool, not a vulnerability.

Chapter 18:
PREVENTION IN ENDOCRINOLOGY

Promoting healthy lifestyles.

Promoting healthy lifestyle habits is like the constant murmur of a gentle melody, reminding us of the importance of looking after our bodies, our minds and our souls. In a modern world where we are besieged by incessant demands, hectic lifestyles and temptations around every corner, it is all the more vital to advocate a return to the fundamentals of health.

1. A balanced diet :
Think of our body as a complex machine that needs the right fuel to function at its best. A diet rich in fruit, vegetables, whole grains, lean proteins and essential fatty acids is essential. Avoiding refined sugars, saturated fats and ultra-processed foods is just as crucial to maintaining an inner balance.

2. Regular physical activity :
Like a rhythmic dance, physical activity is our body's way of expressing its energy, strengthening its resilience and harmonising its functions. Whether it's walking, running, swimming, yoga or any other sport, movement is the key to maintaining optimum health.

3. Rest and sleep :
Like the soothing calm of a starry night, sleep offers us a chance to regenerate, heal and dream. Quality sleep boosts our immune system, improves our mood and boosts our energy.

4. Stress management :
Like a peaceful garden in the middle of a busy city, techniques such as meditation, mindfulness and deep relaxation can help us navigate the storms of life, find our centre and balance our emotions.

5. Healthy relationships :
Human beings are, by nature, social creatures. Cultivating positive relationships, deep friendships and strong family ties is essential to our emotional and psychological well-being.

6. Avoidance of harmful substances :
Just as a purified river is more beneficial than polluted water, avoiding or limiting the consumption of alcohol, tobacco and other drugs protects our bodies from potentially irreversible damage.

7. Continuing education :
The brain, curious and hungry for knowledge, thrives on continuous learning. Whether it's reading, attending lectures or learning a new art, nourishing our minds strengthens our cognitive health.

8. Regular medical check-ups :
Like an architect inspecting the integrity of a structure, medical check-ups can detect anomalies before they become problematic, ensuring early intervention and better management.

Promoting healthy lifestyle habits is much more than just a list of recommendations. It's a philosophy, an invitation to respect, cherish and celebrate our bodies and minds, cultivating daily rituals that uplift, nourish and transform us.

Vaccination and prevention endocrine diseases.

Vaccination is one of the most effective medical interventions for preventing infectious diseases. While endocrine diseases are not in essence infectious diseases and cannot therefore be 'prevented' by vaccination in the traditional sense, certain infections can have an impact on the endocrine system or trigger endocrine disorders. Let's look at this in the wider context of prevention.

1. Vaccination and direct prevention of endocrine disorders :

- **Mumps virus**: Mumps, although mainly associated with inflammation of the salivary glands, can also lead to orchitis (inflammation of the testicles) which, in rare cases, can result in testicular failure.
- **Rubella virus**: If a woman contracts rubella during pregnancy, this can affect the development of the foetus, including the endocrine system.

2. Prevention of conditions that may coexist with endocrine diseases :

- People with diabetes have an increased risk of complications if they contract certain infectious diseases. Vaccination against influenza, pneumonia and hepatitis B is therefore often recommended for diabetics to prevent these infections and their potential complications.

3. Prevention of endocrine autoimmune diseases :

- While the exact cause of most endocrine autoimmune diseases is not yet fully understood, it is known that infections can trigger autoimmune reactions in certain individuals. In this context, preventing infections through vaccination could reduce the risk of developing autoimmune diseases, including those affecting the endocrine system such as Hashimoto's thyroiditis.

4. Long-term impact of infections :
Certain infections can have long-term repercussions on the endocrine system. For example, some studies suggest that viral infections during pregnancy may increase the risk of type 1 diabetes in the child. Although research is ongoing, this underlines the importance of vaccination and infection prevention during this crucial period.
It is also important to note that drugs used to treat certain infections can interact with the endocrine system or with drugs used to treat endocrine disorders. In these cases, preventing infections through vaccination can also help prevent undesirable complications or drug interactions.

Although vaccination is not directly aimed at preventing endocrine diseases, it plays a crucial role in preventing infections that can influence the endocrine system or affect those with endocrine diseases. As with all medical decisions, it is essential to consult a healthcare professional for recommendations specific to each individual.

The educational role of the prevention nurse.

Nurses, at the crossroads of medical care and patient well-being, play a key role in preventing disease and promoting a healthy lifestyle. Their educational role is not limited solely to imparting information, but also encompasses support, advice and guidance to help patients adopt and maintain beneficial health behaviours.

1. Education about the disease :
The nurse provides detailed information about medical conditions, their causes, symptoms, treatments and potential complications. For example, for a diabetic patient,

the nurse will explain the nature of diabetes, variations in blood sugar levels and the importance of monitoring.

2. Self-management skills :
The nurse teaches patients how to manage their disease on a daily basis, such as self-monitoring of blood pressure, injecting insulin or recognising the signs of an asthma attack.

3. Lifestyle advice :
This includes advice on nutrition, exercise, sleep and stress management. For example, advising an obese patient on the importance of a balanced diet and regular physical activity.

4. Prevention of complications :
For patients with chronic illnesses, the nurse will focus on preventing complications. This may include the importance of taking regular medication or following a specific diet.

5. Resources and guidance :
Nurses can refer patients to additional resources, such as support groups, dieticians or therapists.

6. Vaccinations and prophylaxis :
Educate patients about the importance of vaccinations to prevent disease, or prophylactic measures for specific situations, such as preventing malaria when travelling to high-risk areas.

7. Safety and accident prevention :
This can range from preventing falls in the elderly to educating people about the safety of medicines to avoid accidental overdoses.

8. Promoting healthy behaviour :
As well as managing the disease, nurses also promote healthy behaviours, such as stopping smoking, moderate alcohol consumption and regular exercise.

9. Reproductive health education :
Providing information on contraception, health during pregnancy, prevention of STIs and screening tests such as mammography.

10. Emotional and psychological support :
Recognise signs of emotional or psychological distress and offer support, resources or appropriate guidance.

The richness of nurses' educational role lies in their ability to adapt their interventions to each patient, taking into account their individual context, culture, level of education and specific needs. This role goes beyond the simple transmission of information to become a genuine partnership with the patient in his or her healthcare journey.

Collaboration with other health professionals on prevention.

Disease prevention and health promotion are missions that transcend professional boundaries in the medical world. Indeed, inter-professional collaboration is essential if we are to offer holistic and comprehensive care to patients. Let's imagine this collaboration as a symphony where each professional plays his or her own instrument, but all work together to create a harmonious melody.

1. General practitioners and specialists :
They often make the initial diagnosis and create a treatment plan. They also play a pivotal role in coordinating

care, referring patients to other specialists or therapists if necessary.

2. Pharmacists :
They advise patients on the correct use of medicines, drug interactions, side effects and the importance of adherence to treatment. Pharmacists can also offer health screening and vaccinations.

3. Dieticians/nutritionists :
These experts offer advice on diet and nutrition, helping patients to manage diet-related illnesses, lose weight or adopt a specialised diet.

4. Physiotherapists :
They work on physical rehabilitation, helping patients recover from surgery or injury, or manage chronic conditions such as arthritis.

5. Psychologists/psychiatrists :
Mental health is intrinsically linked to physical health. These professionals help patients to manage stress, depression, anxiety or other emotional or mental problems.

6. Public health nurses :
They play a key role in prevention, health promotion and education. They can organise vaccination campaigns, screening tests or educational seminars.

7. Social workers :
They support patients in non-medical areas such as access to care, resolving socio-economic problems or liaising with other community services.

8. Health educators :
These specialists focus on prevention and education, providing information and resources on topics such as

sexual health, smoking prevention and chronic disease management.

9. Physical activity professionals :
Such as kinesiologists or sports trainers, they help patients to adopt and maintain an active lifestyle, adapting exercise programmes to individual needs.

10. Speech therapists and audiologists :
They work respectively on speech and hearing disorders, playing a key role in the prevention, screening and management of these problems.

The collaboration between these various professionals enables a multi-dimensional approach to prevention and care, ensuring that every aspect of a patient's health is taken into account. Like pieces of a complex jigsaw puzzle, each professional brings their own expertise to the table, but it is their joint work that provides a complete and holistic picture of health and wellbeing.

Chapter 19:
ENDOCRINOLOGY AND SURGERY

Preparing the patient
for surgical procedures.

Preparing a patient for surgery is like staging a play. It is essential to ensure that all the elements are in place to guarantee a smooth performance. This preparation encompasses physiological, emotional and logistical aspects, all with the aim of minimising risks and optimising post-operative results.

1. Medical assessment :
Before any surgery, patients undergo a full assessment to determine their suitability for the procedure. This may include blood tests, X-rays or other tests to assess general health and identify any contraindications or risks.

2. Information on the procedure :
It is vital that the patient understands the nature of the operation, its benefits and risks, and what to expect during and after surgery. An open discussion between the surgeon and the patient is essential to enlighten the latter and obtain his or her informed consent.

3. Physical preparation :
> **Fasting**: Patients are often instructed not to eat or drink anything for several hours before surgery to avoid complications from the anaesthetic.
>
> **Hygiene**: A shower with antiseptic soap may be recommended the day before and the day of the operation to minimise the risk of infection.

Medication: Certain medications may need to be stopped or adjusted before the procedure, including anticoagulants or certain supplements.

4. Emotional preparation :
In the face of anxiety or fear, information sessions, support groups or even relaxation techniques can be offered to help patients prepare themselves mentally.

5. Logistics :
Arrival at the hospital: Patients often have to arrive several hours before the operation to prepare for it.
Personal belongings: It is generally advisable to leave valuables at home and bring only the essentials.
Post-operative preparation: This may include organising transport home, setting up a home support system or preparing for a stay in a post-operative care unit.

6. Preparing the surgical site :
The operation site may require specific preparation, such as shaving the hair or marking the area.

7. Discussions with the anaesthetist :
The anaesthetist usually meets the patient before the operation to discuss anaesthetic options, assess the risks and answer any questions.

8. Consent :
Once they have been fully informed, patients sign a consent form confirming their agreement to the procedure.

Preparing the patient for surgery is a crucial step that ensures not only the patient's safety and well-being, but also the success of the operation. Like an orchestra preparing to play, every detail counts, every step is essential to ensure that the symphony of surgery goes off without a hitch.

Post-operative care in endocrinology.

Post-operative care in endocrinology is essential to ensure a successful recovery and avoid complications after surgery. Think of it as a delicate dance between medical care and patient support, where every step is crucial in leading the patient to a safe recovery.

1. Monitoring vital signs :
After any surgery, it is vital to monitor the patient's blood pressure, heart rate, temperature and respiratory rate regularly for any abnormal signs.

2. Monitoring hormone levels :
In endocrinology, it is crucial to monitor hormone levels, particularly if the surgery involves glands such as the thyroid, parathyroid or adrenal glands. Hormonal imbalances may require immediate medical intervention.

3. Pain management :
Pain is a common concern after surgery. Analgesic drugs will be prescribed, and it is essential to ensure that the patient receives adequate analgesia without suffering undesirable side effects.

4. Monitoring the surgical wound :
Inspect the wound regularly for signs of infection, bleeding or other complications. It is also important to advise the patient on home care of the wound.

5. Rehabilitation and physiotherapy :
In some cases, exercises or physiotherapy sessions may be recommended to help functional recovery.

6. Nutritional monitoring :
Depending on the surgery, specific nutritional recommendations may be necessary, particularly if the surgery affects the patient's ability to eat normally.

7. Patient education :
It is essential to inform the patient about post-operative care, the signs of complications to look out for and the stages of recovery. This may also include information on medication, hormone adjustments and follow-up appointments.

8. Emotional and psychological support :
Surgery can have an emotional impact on the patient. Offering support, resources and, if necessary, referral to mental health professionals can help patients manage this stress.

9. Scheduling follow-up appointments :
Post-operative visits are essential to monitor recovery, adjust medication or treatments and address any concerns the patient may have.

10. Long-term assessment :
In endocrinology, the consequences of surgery may require long-term monitoring of hormone levels and glandular functions.

Post-operative care in endocrinology is a harmony between medical science, the art of care and compassion. Each patient is unique, and care must be tailored to their specific needs, ensuring not only physical recovery but also emotional and psychological well-being.

Working with the surgical team.

Working with the surgical team is like a well-orchestrated choreography, where each member knows his or her role, moves with precision and complements the movements of the others. Everyone, from the surgeon to the nurse to the anaesthetist, plays their part.

The surgical team is more than just the surgeon, although he or she is often at the heart of the action. The surgeon is the architect of the operation, with the vision and skills to perform what are often delicate procedures. However, without the close collaboration of the other members of the team, his work would be far more complex.

The anaesthetist, for example, is the patient's guardian during the operation, ensuring that the patient is both pain-free and safe, constantly monitoring vital signs and adjusting medication to ensure a stable anaesthetic.

Operating theatre nurses, with their in-depth knowledge of surgical instruments and procedures, anticipate the surgeon's needs, handing over the right tools at the right time and ensuring that the operating field remains sterile. They are the link between the surgeon, the equipment and the patient, ensuring that the surgery runs smoothly.

Then there are the technicians and assistants, whose role, although less visible, is just as crucial. They prepare the operating theatre, make sure all the equipment is ready and working, and often help out during the procedure.
Once the operation is over, it's the turn of the recovery room nurses to take over, monitoring the patient as they emerge from anaesthesia, ensuring a smooth transition from unconsciousness to full consciousness and looking after their comfort and safety.

Collaboration with the surgical team is a demonstration of the power of synergy. When everyone works in harmony, with clear communication and shared goals, the patient is assured of the best possible care. And although each member of the team has his or her own dance to perform, it is their collective movement, this harmonious, interconnected dance, that creates the magic of modern medicine.

Rehabilitation and return to normal.

Rehabilitation and the return to normality after an operation or illness are essential stages in the healing process, rather like the final act of a play, when the protagonist finds his or her way to resolution and renewal. It's not just a question of physical healing, but also of mental and emotional adaptation to regain one's previous rhythm of life.
The rehabilitation process begins as soon as you leave the hospital bed. For some, this means regaining the strength to walk after a long period of immobilisation; for others, it may involve more in-depth re-education to regain motor or cognitive functions. Physiotherapists, occupational therapists and other professionals may be called in to guide patients through specific exercises and therapies tailored to their needs.

However, the process of returning to normality does not stop with physical recovery. Often, a period of disability or illness can lead to feelings of vulnerability, frustration or sadness. It is therefore crucial to address these emotional aspects too. Sessions with psychologists, support groups or counsellors can help patients to manage these emotions and regain their self-confidence.

Returning to everyday life can also require a period of adjustment. Returning to work, managing household chores, looking after the family or simply getting back into social life are all challenges that can seem overwhelming at first. It can be helpful for the patient to gradually resume these activities, to set achievable goals and to celebrate each small victory.

Relatives also play a crucial role in rehabilitation and the return to normality. Their support, patience and encouragement can do much to ease the patient's transition. Their involvement can range from simply listening to the patient to assisting with daily activities or taking part in family therapy.

Finally, the return to normal is also a period of prevention. Patients may be encouraged to adopt a healthier lifestyle, undergo regular medical check-ups or take medication to prevent recurrence of the disease or other complications.

Rehabilitation and the return to normality are journeys that are as much physical as they are emotional. Like the denouement of a story, it is a period of resolution, learning and hope, when patients rediscover their place in the world, strengthened by the trials they have been through and supported by the people around them.

Chapter 20:
ENDOCRINOLOGY AND OTHER MEDICAL SPECIALITIES

Collaboration with cardiology.

Collaboration between endocrinology and cardiology is like an alliance between two virtuosos, each an expert in their own field, but working in harmony to interpret a complex melody: the patient's overall health. These two medical disciplines, although distinct, frequently intersect, as hormonal imbalances can have repercussions on the heart, and vice versa.

Imagine the human body as a web woven of interdependent relationships. The heart, that powerful pump, is influenced by many factors, including the hormones produced in different parts of the body. Conversely, the functioning of our endocrine organs can be directly affected by the health of our cardiovascular system.

1. Diabetes and heart disease :
One of the most obvious examples of this collaboration is the link between diabetes and heart disease. Diabetic patients are at increased risk of developing cardiovascular disease. As a result, joint monitoring by endocrinologists and cardiologists can optimise management and prevent complications.

2. Thyroid and heart function :
Thyroid disorders, such as hyperthyroidism, can lead to arrhythmias or other heart problems. Close collaboration between the two specialists guarantees comprehensive care and accurate risk assessment.

3. Hormones and hypertension :
Conditions such as Cushing's syndrome or a pheochromocytoma tumour can lead to hypertension. The role of the cardiologist in monitoring blood pressure and treatment is essential, while working with the endocrinologist to treat the underlying cause.

4. Drugs and interactions :
Some endocrine drugs can have cardiac side effects, and cardiac drugs can influence endocrine function. Open communication between specialists is therefore crucial to balancing therapies.

5. Search and advanced :
The two disciplines also collaborate on research, studying the links between hormones and heart disease, or exploring new treatments for common conditions.

6. Patient education :
Providing patients with holistic education on how their heart and endocrine systems interact strengthens their involvement in their own health, enabling them to adopt healthier lifestyle choices.

The collaboration between endocrinology and cardiology is a delicate dance, a medical symbiosis. Together, these disciplines ensure that the heart and hormones, although operating to their own rhythms, play a harmonious melody for the overall well-being of the patient.

Interaction with nephrology.

The interaction between endocrinology and nephrology is an essential alliance, like two musicians playing a duet, complementing and enriching each other's melodies. The kidneys, the central organs of nephrology, play a crucial role in many bodily functions, including balancing fluids, filtering waste products and regulating various hormones. These functions make them intimately involved in many aspects of endocrinology.

1. Diabetes and kidney disease :

Diabetes is one of the main causes of kidney failure. The kidneys can be damaged by excess sugar in the blood, leading to diabetic nephropathy. In this context, endocrinologists and nephrologists often work hand in hand to monitor and treat patients.

2. Hypertension and the kidneys :

Hypertension can be both a cause and a consequence of kidney disease. Hormones such as aldosterone, which is regulated by the adrenal glands (a field of endocrinology), play a key role **in the regulation of blood pressure by the kidneys.**

3. Parathyroid gland disorders :

The parathyroid glands, which regulate calcium in the blood, interact closely with the kidneys. Disorders such as hyperparathyroidism can have repercussions on renal function, requiring close collaboration between endocrinologists and nephrologists.

4. Medicines and kidneys :

Many drugs used in endocrinology are metabolised or excreted by the kidneys. The nephrologist therefore plays a crucial role in the dosage and monitoring of these drugs in patients with reduced renal function.

5. Joint research :

The interactions between the endocrine and renal systems offer numerous opportunities for research. Joint studies can lead to a better understanding of diseases and to new therapeutic strategies.

6. Education and prevention :

Given the close relationship between hormonal imbalances and kidney disease, educating patients about prevention is fundamental. By understanding how sugar, blood pressure or electrolyte imbalances can impact their kidneys, patients are better equipped to manage their health.

The collaboration between endocrinology and nephrology is a perfect demonstration of how medicine is interconnected. As in an orchestra, each section, although playing its own notes, contributes to the overall symphony. By working together, these two specialities offer optimal care and a harmonious melody for patients' health.

Relations with gynaecology and andrology.

Endocrinology, gynaecology and andrology form a medical triptych closely intertwined around the mysteries and wonders of the human endocrine system. Like waves on an ocean, hormones shape and influence the landscape of reproduction and sexual health, making collaboration between these specialities not only logical but essential.

1. Reproduction and fertility :
Infertility, whether male or female, is often the result of a hormonal imbalance. Whether it's ovulatory abnormalities in women or problems with sperm production in men, endocrinologists play a key role in diagnosing, understanding and treating these disorders, working closely with gynaecologists and andrologists.

2. Polycystic ovary syndrome (PCOS) :
This endocrine disorder, common in women of childbearing age, presents a variety of symptoms ranging from menstrual irregularities to infertility. A collaborative approach between endocrinologist and gynaecologist is essential for holistic management.

3. Gender transition :
Transgender people may require hormonal interventions as part of their transition. In this delicate process, the endocrinologist works alongside specialists in gynaecology and andrology to ensure a smooth and safe transition.

4. Menopause and andropause :
These natural phases of life, marked by hormonal changes, are managed jointly by endocrinologists and gynaecologists for women, and by endocrinologists and andrologists for men, guaranteeing appropriate and comprehensive support.

5. Glandular tumours and disorders :
Some disorders of the reproductive glands, such as ovarian or testicular tumours, may be hormonal in origin. In these cases, collaboration between the various specialities is essential for accurate diagnosis and optimal treatment.

6. Hormonal contraception :
The endocrinologist, together with the gynaecologist, is often involved in the choice and monitoring of hormonal contraceptive methods, ensuring the optimum balance for the woman's health.

7. Sexual disorders :
Endocrinologists are often involved in libido disorders and other sexual dysfunctions, working closely with gynaecologists and andrologists to provide comprehensive patient care.

The beauty of medicine lies in its ability to transcend specialities, to establish connections between seemingly distinct fields to offer holistic care. The interaction between endocrinology, gynaecology and andrology is a harmonious dance of specialists, each bringing their own expertise, but all working together for the ultimate well-being of the patient.

Interface with psychiatry and psychology.

The interface between endocrinology and the disciplines of psychiatry and psychology is a fascinating convergence of body and mind. Like the notes of a complex melody, hormones influence our mood, emotions and cognition, while our thoughts, feelings and experiences can, in turn, affect our hormonal balance. This two-way interaction reveals the profound intertwining of our physiology with our psyche.

1. Impact of hormonal imbalances on mood :
Conditions such as hypothyroidism or hyperthyroidism can lead to symptoms such as depression or anxiety. In such cases, a combined approach between the endocrinologist and the psychiatrist or psychologist is essential for holistic management.

2. Stress and the endocrine system :
The stress response is mediated by hormones, in particular cortisol. Chronic stress can upset hormonal balance, and vice versa. By working together, specialists can better understand and manage this dynamic relationship.

3. Eating disorders :
Illnesses such as anorexia and bulimia have both psychological and endocrine components. The joint work of the endocrinologist and psychiatrist can offer essential support to these patients.

4. Infertility and emotional well-being :
Infertility can have a major impact on the emotional well-being of an individual or couple. Alongside hormonal

treatments, psychological support can be crucial in helping patients deal with stress, frustration and grief.

5. Gender transition :
Beyond the hormonal aspect of transition, transgender people may need psychological support to navigate the social, emotional and mental challenges associated with their journey.

6. Chronic endocrine diseases :
Living with a chronic illness such as diabetes can be psychologically challenging. Working with mental health professionals can help patients manage the emotional and behavioural aspects of their illness.

7. Neuropsychiatric syndromes :
Some syndromes, such as Cushing's syndrome, have both endocrine and neuropsychiatric manifestations. Joint management ensures better understanding and comprehensive intervention.

The interaction between endocrinology, psychiatry and psychology is a revelation of the interdependence of body and mind. It is a delicate dance where physiology meets the psyche, and where mutual respect and collaboration between specialists are essential if we are to offer comprehensive care that is truly patient-centred.

Chapter 21:
MANAGING DIFFICULT AND CONFLICTUAL SITUATIONS

Managing conflict with patients and their families.

Navigating the sometimes turbulent waters of medicine requires not only clinical expertise, but also communication and empathy skills. Conflicts with patients and their families can arise for a variety of reasons, from differences of opinion about treatments, to frustrations with the care system, to emotions heightened by illness. Managing these situations is an art in itself, a delicate dance between validating feelings, mediating and preserving medical ethics.

1. Active listening :
Every patient's story is unique, and every emotion is valid. Listening actively, without interrupting or judging, can often defuse a tense situation. Hearing and validating the concerns of the patient or their family is the first step in establishing common ground.

2. Transparent communication :
Most conflicts arise from misunderstandings or a lack of clarity. Open, honest and clear communication, explaining the reasons for medical decisions and clarifying uncertainties, can reduce tensions.

3. Empathy :
Acknowledging and validating the patient's or family's emotions is essential. Sometimes a simple "I understand this is difficult for you" can make a big difference.

4. Negotiation :
Finding an acceptable compromise is sometimes necessary. This may involve discussing different treatment options, exploring alternatives or considering a second opinion.

5. Involving intermediaries :
In particularly tense situations, involving mediators such as social workers, counsellors or patient advocates can help facilitate communication and find solutions.

6. Education :
Ignorance or lack of knowledge can fuel fears and conflict. Providing relevant information, in the form of brochures, videos or education sessions, can help patients and families to better understand the situation.

7. Self-reflection :
It is crucial for healthcare professionals to reflect on their own behaviour and communication. Did my language, tone or actions contribute to the conflict? How can I improve?

8. Establish clear limits :
While empathy and understanding are essential, it is also crucial to maintain a certain professional authority and establish clear limits, especially if the patient's or family's behaviour becomes abusive.

9. Support among colleagues :
Discussing difficult situations with colleagues can offer a different perspective, advice or simply emotional support.

Medicine is more than a science; it is a human art, involving complex relationships, emotions and dynamics. Managing conflict with patients and their families therefore requires an equally nuanced approach, combining clinical skill, communication, empathy and resilience.

Collaboration
in a sometimes tense environment.

Working in the medical sector can often be likened to walking a tightrope. High-pressure situations, urgency, fear, uncertainty and strong emotions are part of everyday life. In such tense environments, effective collaboration is both a challenge and a necessity. But, like the instruments of an orchestra that find harmony even in the midst of a tumultuous symphony, healthcare professionals can align to deliver exceptional care.

1. Clear communication :
In a tense environment, every second counts. Concise, clear and direct communication is essential to ensure effective coordination.

2. Mutual trust :
Trust is the cornerstone of any collaboration. Each member of the team must have confidence in the competence and judgement of the others, in the knowledge that every decision is taken in the patient's best interests.
3. Understanding roles :
Each healthcare professional has a unique role. Understanding each other's responsibilities and competencies makes for smoother collaboration and avoids overlaps or oversights.

4. Emotional regulation :
Learning to manage your emotions and remain calm and centred, even in the most stressful situations, is essential. This not only improves decision-making, but also creates a sense of stability within the team.

5. Constructive feedback :
Even in moments of high tension, it is important to give and receive feedback. This feedback, when given

constructively, can lead to rapid improvements and avoid future mistakes.

6. Regular debriefings :
After particularly stressful or complicated situations, it's a good idea to get together for a debriefing. This allows us to analyse what went well and what could be improved, and to process any residual emotions.

7. Further training :
Regular training sessions, focusing on collaboration and communication, can strengthen team spirit and provide tools to better manage tense situations.

8. Emotional support :
Offering emotional support to colleagues, whether it's a simple word of encouragement, a sympathetic ear or a shoulder to lean on, strengthens team cohesion.

9. Mutual respect :
Recognising the value and contribution of each team member, whatever their position or specialism, is fundamental to maintaining a collaborative environment.
Collaborating in a tense environment is a bit like dancing in the middle of a storm. There will be moments of uncertainty, hesitant steps and mistakes. But with clear communication, mutual respect and unwavering support, the team can synchronise, evolve in harmony and get through even the most complex situations with grace and skill.

Navigating emotionally charged situations.

Navigating emotionally charged situations is a challenge intrinsic to medicine and many other fields. These moments, imbued with pain, fear, uncertainty or tension, require a gentle yet firm approach, a blend of deep empathy and unwavering professionalism. It's like going through a storm at sea; each wave of emotion needs to be recognised and approached with care to ensure safe navigation.

1. Emotion recognition :
The first step in navigating an emotionally charged situation is to recognise the emotions present, whether they are those of the patient, their family, or even their own. Accepting that these feelings are natural and valid creates a space for mutual understanding.

2. Active listening :
Offering an attentive ear, without interrupting or judging, can often ease tension. Active listening shows patients and their families that their feelings are heard and respected.

3. Validation :
A simple "I understand that this is difficult for you" or "Your feelings are completely valid" can bring immense comfort. Validating emotions does not necessarily mean that you agree, but that you recognise the other person's feelings.

4. Keep calm:
In a tumultuous sea of emotions, the healthcare professional must be the lighthouse, radiating calm and stability. Taking deep breaths, practising mindfulness and remembering to stay centred can help maintain this serenity.

5. Use clear, soothing language:
Choosing your words carefully, avoiding medical jargon and using a soothing tone, can facilitate communication and reduce anxiety.

6. Setting limits :
While empathy and understanding are essential, it is also important to establish clear boundaries, especially if the patient or family becomes aggressive or abusive.

7. Asking for help :
If the situation becomes too difficult to manage alone, don't hesitate to ask a colleague, supervisor or even a mental health professional for support or mediation.

8. Self-reflection :
After navigating an emotional situation, take a moment to reflect. How does it make you feel? Is there anything you could have done differently? Self-reflection is a powerful tool for personal and professional growth.

9. Emotional support :
Take care of yourself. Dealing with emotionally charged situations can leave an emotional residue. Talking to colleagues, consulting a counsellor or practising relaxation techniques can help you manage this stress.

Navigating the rough waters of emotional situations is undoubtedly one of the most demanding, but also one of the most rewarding, challenges of the medical profession. It's at these moments that you can really touch someone's life, bring comfort in the midst of pain, and be the lighthouse in the storm.

Resources and support for nurses in difficult situations.

Nurses, like many other healthcare professionals, are often confronted with intense and emotionally challenging situations. These moments can leave lasting impressions, sometimes leading to burnout, anxiety or even depression.

Yet at the heart of these challenges lie opportunities for growth, support and resilience. Here's how nurses can find resources and support to navigate these tumultuous waters.

1. Clinical supervision :
Supervision provides nurses with a space to discuss difficult cases, share concerns and seek advice. It's an opportunity to learn, reflect and grow professionally in a supportive environment.

2. Support groups :
Joining or forming a support group for nurses can be incredibly beneficial. These groups provide a platform for sharing experiences, coping strategies and resources.

3. Individual therapy :
Some nurses may benefit from individual therapy to deal with particularly traumatic experiences or to manage personal problems that interfere with their work.

4. Stress management training :
Workshops or training in stress management techniques, such as mindfulness, meditation or progressive relaxation, can help nurses to manage the tensions inherent in their profession.

5. Online resources :
There are many forums, blogs and websites dedicated to supporting nurses. These platforms can offer advice, testimonials and resources to help nurses through difficult times.

6. Mentoring :
More experienced nurses can offer valuable support to novices as mentors, sharing their experiences, knowledge and coping strategies.

7. Work-life balance :
It's essential to take time for yourself, recharge your batteries and reconnect with activities and passions outside work. This balance can help prevent burnout and renew energy.

8. Employee assistance services :
Many hospitals and medical institutions offer employee assistance services, which can provide a range of resources from counselling to financial or legal advice.

9. Further training :
Continuing education and training can boost nurses' confidence, help them feel more competent in the face of challenges and give them new tools to manage difficult situations.

10. Professional networking :
Attending conferences, workshops and professional events can not only broaden nurses' knowledge and skills, but also give them the opportunity to meet colleagues, share experiences and build a support network.

Working as a nurse is both a challenge and a blessing. It's a job where you touch people's lives, where every day is a new opportunity to bring healing, comfort and hope. But it's also a demanding job that requires support, resources and constant attention to one's own well-being.

Chapter 22:
THE FUTURE OF TRAINING
IN ENDOCRINOLOGY

Educational developments
and training formats.

Over time, education has undergone countless transformations, shaped by technological advances, changing social needs, and discoveries in pedagogy. While education used to be primarily about the one-way transmission of knowledge, pedagogical developments have since embraced more interactive, personalised and learner-centred methods.

The traditional classroom, with its rows of desks facing a dominant teacher, has gradually given way to more flexible and collaborative learning spaces. Round tables, modular spaces and technologically equipped environments now encourage discussion, teamwork and a more holistic approach to education.

With the advent of digital technology, training formats have also undergone a revolution. Online courses, whether MOOCs or specialist learning platforms, have democratised access to education, allowing anyone with an internet connection to immerse themselves in a multitude of subjects. These formats have not only made it easier to learn at your own pace, but have also introduced innovative teaching methods such as serious games, virtual reality and simulation.

Project and problem-based learning has also challenged the traditional model of memorisation and recitation. Rather than focusing on the pure retention of information, this approach places the emphasis on solving concrete problems, applying knowledge and developing skills such as critical thinking, creativity and collaboration.

But beyond the formats and methods, it is the underlying philosophy of education that has evolved. We have moved from seeing education as preparation for life, to education as life itself. The learning journey is no longer seen as a straight line leading from point A to point B, but rather as a spiral journey, where learning is continuous, iterative and adapted to the changing needs of the individual.

So, as we contemplate today's educational developments and training formats, we can't help but marvel at the wealth of learning opportunities available to us. Education, in its perpetual quest for improvement, innovation and adaptation, continues to reinvent itself, testifying to its central role in the evolution of our society.

The role of simulation in training.

Simulation, once relegated to the confines of specialist vocational training, has now risen to the forefront of modern education. It offers a bridge between theory and practice, a space where error, far from being punitive, becomes a valuable learning opportunity.
Imagine a medical student who, before even touching a patient, can perform a complex surgical operation on a hyper-realistic mannequin, or a pilot who confronts emergency situations in the virtual cockpit of a simulator before taking the controls of a real aircraft. This is the power of simulation: it creates a safe, controlled environment where learners can acquire skills, make decisions and, above all, learn from their mistakes without any real consequences.

But simulation goes far beyond these obvious examples. Thanks to technological advances, it has infiltrated a variety of fields. Corporate role-playing games, for example, simulate professional situations to develop communication or negotiation skills. In architecture, students can use virtual reality to 'walk' through structures they have designed, assessing aesthetics and functionality before the first shovel is turned.

What makes simulation so rich is its adaptability. It can be as simple as a role-playing game or as complex as a fully immersive reconstruction using augmented reality. Whatever its form, it meets a fundamental need in education: to transform passive knowledge into active skills.

One of the main advantages of simulation is that it places the learner at the heart of the learning process. It's no longer a question of passively memorising information, but of actively participating, making decisions, interacting and experimenting. Simulation makes learning tangible, concrete and rooted in reality, even if it is reconstructed.
However, like any teaching method, simulation has its limits. It requires resources, from expensive equipment to the expertise needed to create realistic scenarios. What's more, it can never perfectly reproduce the complexity and unpredictability of the real world. However, when used properly, simulation remains an invaluable tool, a springboard that enables learners to move from theory to practice with confidence and skill.

In the age of digital technology, where information is abundant but experience is often limited, simulation is establishing itself as a pillar of modern training, reminding us that sometimes the best way to learn is to do, even if it's in a reconstructed world.

Self-training and new technologies.

In the continuous flow of the digital age, where knowledge is just a click away, self-learning, fuelled by new technologies, is emerging as a beacon guiding learners towards as yet unexplored horizons. Learning is no longer strictly confined to the walls of a classroom or the pages of a textbook. It is dynamic, interactive, and above all, it adapts to the pace of each individual.

Self-learning, as the name suggests, is a process whereby individuals take charge of their own learning. And on this journey, new technologies are the ideal companion. E-learning platforms, MOOCs (Massive Open Online Courses), educational podcasts, specialist forums and even YouTube videos are all resources that have transformed the way we learn, making education more accessible and customisable.

The power of new technologies lies in their ability to break down the traditional barriers of education. Would you like to learn programming at midnight? Or follow a Harvard astrophysics course from the comfort of your own living room? It's all possible. These tools offer unprecedented flexibility, allowing learners to choose what they want to study, when and how.

Technologies have also enhanced the interactive aspect of learning. With simulations, educational games and even virtual reality, the learner is no longer a mere spectator, but becomes a player in his or her training. This interactivity, combined with the immediacy of feedback, means that learning can be adapted and adjusted in real time, maximising the effectiveness of each study session.

But self-directed learning, while emancipating, also has its challenges. Without a clear framework, motivation can wane. The abundance of information can also be overwhelming, making it difficult to distinguish between reliable sources and less rigorous content. What's more, the lack of direct human interaction can, for some, make the experience isolating.

Nevertheless, these challenges in no way detract from the revolutionary potential of new technologies in self-learning. In fact, they underline the importance of a balanced approach, where technological tools are complemented by moments of reflection, discussion and exchange with others.

Self-learning in the digital age is a delicate dance between the individual and technology. It invites curiosity and autonomy, while reminding us of the importance of community and sharing. In this ever-changing landscape, one thing remains certain: learning is a never-ending journey, and thanks to new technologies, the road is more exciting than ever.

The importance of feedback and continuing education.

The acquisition of knowledge never really ends at the end of an initial training course or an academic curriculum. On the contrary, working life, with all its challenges, innovations and changes, is a constant reminder that learning is a continuous process. In this context, feedback and continuous training are two essential pillars of this perpetual quest for improvement and adaptation.

Feedback, by capturing the lessons learned from past situations, whether successes or failures, is invaluable. It offers a retrospective vision, a mirror in which individuals and organisations can reflect on themselves, identify areas for improvement and consolidate good practice. It's an introspective approach that turns every situation into a learning opportunity. By avoiding the repetition of past mistakes and capitalising on successes, REX encourages sustained professional and organisational growth.

Continuing education is a proactive response to a constantly changing world. With technological advances, market developments and socio-cultural changes, it is vital for professionals to stay up to date, acquire new skills and adapt to the changing realities of their profession. Continuing education is not just about upgrading skills; it is an expression of professional curiosity, a desire to excel and to remain relevant in a competitive environment.

The interaction between these two pillars, feedback and ongoing training, is synergetic. Feedback often guides training needs, by identifying gaps or areas requiring reinforcement. Conversely, continuous training, by exposing professionals to new methods, technologies or practices, can generate new feedback, fuelling a virtuous cycle of continuous improvement.

It should be stressed that humility and open-mindedness are paramount in this process. Accepting criticism, admitting mistakes and embracing change requires professional maturity. It's an invitation to see beyond the ego, to recognise that learning is a journey, not a destination.
Ultimately, feedback and ongoing training remind us that professionalism is not a static quality. It is a dynamic, a commitment to evolve, grow and adapt. In a world where change is the only constant, this commitment to learning and developing is more than a necessity; it's an imperative.

Chapter 23:
FUTURE PROSPECTS AND INNOVATIONS

The changing role of the nurse in endocrinology.

Endocrinology, the branch of medicine focusing on the endocrine glands and hormones, has undergone profound changes over the last few decades. In parallel with these advances, the role of the endocrinology nurse has also changed, expanding their skills and responsibilities within this medical speciality.

Historically, the endocrinology nurse was mainly responsible for basic clinical tasks: administering medication, monitoring vital signs and educating patients about their condition. But with time and advances in medical science, this limited vision has evolved into a much more comprehensive and versatile role.

One of the first notable developments was the development and mastery of techniques specific to endocrinology. For example, the management of insulin pumps and continuous glucose monitors has become an essential skill for nurses working with diabetic patients.

In addition, the educational role of nurses has been considerably strengthened. Therapeutic education, based on teaching patients about the specifics of their disease, their treatment and self-monitoring measures, has become central. This approach aims to make patients more autonomous, enabling them to better understand their illness and act accordingly to preserve their health.

Technological developments have also had an impact on the profession. With the advent of telemedicine, endocrinology nurses can now monitor patients remotely, providing advice and support without the constraints of a physical consultation.

What's more, the role of the nurse has been extended to include coordinating care. They are often the interface between the patient, the endocrinologist and other healthcare professionals such as dieticians, chiropodists and psychologists. This coordinating role is particularly crucial in the management of chronic diseases such as diabetes, where a multidisciplinary approach is essential.

Finally, the psychological and emotional dimension of the nurse's role has been affirmed. Endocrine diseases, with their potential impact on aspects as varied as growth, reproduction and metabolism, can have profound repercussions on patients' quality of life. The endocrinology nurse is on the front line, providing psychological support, listening, reassuring and, if necessary, guiding.

The changing role of the endocrinology nurse reflects the growing complexity and richness of this medical speciality. The nurse has gone from being a simple operator to becoming a fully-fledged health player, essential to the overall, individualised care of the endocrine patient.

New technologies and their impact.

At the dawn of the 21st century, new technologies, through their disruptive innovations, have shaped almost every aspect of our daily lives, influencing our behaviour, changing our societies and redefining entire industries.

Their impact is multidimensional, oscillating between undeniable advantages and unprecedented challenges.

1. Communication:
Social networking, instant messaging and video platforms have revolutionised the way we communicate. We are now connected to a global network, able to interact in real time with someone on the other side of the world. This has facilitated the sharing of information, international collaboration and the rapid dissemination of ideas. However, it has also given rise to problems of misinformation, cyberbullying and virtual isolation.

2. Education:
E-learning, MOOCs and interactive educational tools have made education accessible to millions of people. Geographical and financial barriers are gradually being removed. Nevertheless, this raises questions about the value of the traditional diploma, the homogeneity of teaching and the risk of disparities in the quality of education.

3. Cheers:
Telemedicine, genomics, connected objects and artificial intelligence in medicine have revolutionised diagnosis, treatment and patient monitoring. However, this raises concerns about privacy, data security and ethics.
4. Work:
Digitalisation, automation and artificial intelligence have optimised many processes, making some jobs obsolete while creating new ones. While this promises greater efficiency, it also raises concerns about job security, lifelong learning and job insecurity.

5. Leisure activities:
Video games, virtual reality and streaming platforms have enriched our entertainment. These innovations offer new immersive experiences, but they are also sparking debate

about technological dependency, the impact on mental health and the dilution of traditional culture.

6. Environment:
While technology has contributed to certain environmental problems, it is also an essential part of the solution. Innovations in renewable energy, waste management and sustainable agriculture could be the key to combating climate change.

7. The company:
New technologies have redefined our social relationships, our concept of privacy and even our perception of reality. They have enabled a global movement towards greater transparency, but have also fuelled debates about surveillance, societal polarisation and the influence of technology giants.

The impact of new technologies is both fascinating and complex. While they hold incredible potential to improve the human condition, they require careful thought, regulation and rigorous ethics to ensure that they benefit everyone, without compromising our values or our humanity.

Clinical research : an opportunity for nurses.

Clinical research is at the heart of medical advances, constantly seeking to improve care, treatments and interventions to ensure a better quality of life for patients. Nurses, being on the front line of patient care, are ideally placed to become actively involved in this field. Clinical research presents a multitude of opportunities for nurses, both for their professional development and for improving care.

1. Contribution to science and quality of care :
Nurses have a deep and unique understanding of patient needs, care dynamics and clinical challenges. By participating in research, they can help create new knowledge, influence clinical protocols and contribute to more informed, patient-centred care.

2. Career development :
Clinical research offers nurses the opportunity to diversify their careers. They can become nurse researchers, clinical study coordinators or specialist consultants. This enables them to acquire new skills, such as scientific writing, project management and biostatistics.

3. Impact on health policy :
With empirical data, nurses can influence decision-makers, advocate evidence-based health policies and promote changes in health systems.

4. Interprofessional collaboration :
Clinical research strengthens collaboration between different healthcare professionals. Nurses can work with doctors, pharmacists, statisticians and other specialists, promoting a multidisciplinary approach to clinical problems.

5. Autonomy and leadership :
Participation in research reinforces the nurse's role as a leader in healthcare. It positions nurses as key contributors to medical science and highlights the value of their perspective in the research process.

6. Education and training :
Involvement in clinical research enables nurses to remain at the cutting edge of medical knowledge. They can also become trainers or lecturers, sharing their findings with colleagues or the next generation of nurses.

7. Job satisfaction :
Taking part in discovering new interventions, improving care or resolving clinical challenges can bring great professional satisfaction. It's an opportunity for nurses to see first-hand the impact of their work on patients' lives.

Clinical research is a field rich in opportunities for nurses. It allows them to develop professionally, improve patient care and make a significant contribution to medical science and public health. In an ever-changing medical world, nurses' involvement in clinical research is more essential than ever.

Conclusion:
THE IMPORTANCE OF DEDICATION, EMPATHY AND COMPETENCE IN CARE ENDOCRINE PATIENTS.

In the vast world of medicine, caring for patients with endocrine disorders is a delicate task that requires more than just technical skills. The patient's journey through the labyrinth of hormones and glands is often marked by intense emotions, uncertainties and a quest for balance. So dedication, empathy and skill are three essential pillars in supporting these patients with respect and efficiency.

Dedication is the solid anchor that keeps nurses at the service of the patient's well-being. These disorders, which are often chronic, require prolonged attention, where monitoring, adaptability and constant commitment become crucial. Endocrine patients can go through an emotional and physiological rollercoaster, and the nurse's dedication ensures a constant, reassuring and determined presence every step of the way.

However, pure skill is not enough. Empathy, the ability to put yourself in the patient's shoes, to feel and understand their emotions, is the light that illuminates the path. Hormonal imbalances can have a profound impact on mood, self-perception and quality of life. In the face of this, empathy provides a safe space where the patient feels heard, validated and understood. It is in this space that emotional healing can begin, alongside medical interventions.

And of course, at the heart of it all is expertise. Endocrine disorders are complex, interconnected and require in-depth knowledge for appropriate management. Every patient is unique, and their response to treatment can vary considerably. Competence ensures that the nurse is not only well informed, but also able to use this knowledge adaptively, tailoring care to the specific needs of each patient.

When these three pillars - dedication, empathy and competence - combine harmoniously, they form the trinity of authentic care. For the endocrine patient, this means being treated with dignity, receiving quality care and feeling supported every step of the way, whatever the challenges encountered. In the delicate world of endocrinology, these three qualities are not just desirable; they are essential to providing truly holistic care.

Glossary of medical terms.

The medical field is rich in specific terminology. Here is a simplified glossary of some commonly used medical terms. Note that this list is far from exhaustive, and it is recommended that you consult specialist medical sources for a more detailed definition.

A

- **Anemia:** Reduction in the number of red blood cells in the blood.
- **Antibiotic:** Drug used to treat bacterial infections.
- **Aseptic:** Absence of pathogenic micro-organisms.

B

- **Biopsy:** removal of a small sample of tissue for microscopic examination.
- **Bronchitis:** Inflammation of the bronchial tubes.

C

- **Cardiology:** Study of the heart and its diseases.
- **Surgery:** Medical practice involving manual and instrumental interventions on a patient.
- **Cyanosis:** Bluish discolouration of the skin due to a lack of oxygen.

D

- **Diabetes: A** disease characterised by insufficient insulin production or poor use of insulin by the body.
- **Dialysis:** Blood purification process for people suffering from kidney failure.

E

- **Ultrasound:** Imaging technique using sound waves to create images of internal organs.
- **Endocrinology:** Study of the endocrine glands and hormones.

F

- **Fibrosis:** Excessive formation of fibrous tissue in an organ.

Fracture: Breakage or fracture of a bone.

G

Gastroenterology: Study of the stomach and intestine.
Genome: The complete DNA of an organism.

H

Hematology: Study of blood and blood disorders.
Hypertension: High blood pressure.

I

Immunology: Study of the immune system.
Infection: Invasion and multiplication of pathogenic micro-organisms in the body.

J

Jaundice: yellowing of the skin due to an accumulation of bilirubin.

K

Cyst: abnormal mass containing liquid or semi-solid material.

L

Leukaemia: Blood cancer affecting white blood cells.

M

Mammography: X-ray of the breast.
Metabolism: All the chemical reactions occurring in a living organism.

N

Neurology: Study of the nervous system.
Nephrology: Study of the kidneys.

O

Oncology: Study of tumours and cancer.
Osteoporosis: Reduction in bone density, making bones brittle.

P

Paediatrics: Branch of medicine dealing with children.
Pharmacology: Study of drugs and their effects.

Q

- **Quadrant:** One of four equal parts of an area or surface.

R

- **Radiology: The** study of X-rays to diagnose and treat disease.
- **Rheumatology:** Study of joint diseases.

S

- **Serum:** The liquid part of the blood without the cells.
- **Symptom:** Manifestation of an illness experienced by the patient.

T

- **Thrombosis:** Formation of a blood clot inside a blood vessel.
- **Toxicology:** Study of poisons and toxins.

U

- **Urology:** Study of the kidneys, ureters, bladder and urethra.
- **Ulcer:** Open wound on the skin or mucous membrane.

V

- **Vaccination:** Administration of a vaccine to induce immunity against a specific disease.
- **Virology:** Study of viruses.

W

- WBC (White Blood Cells): White blood cells.

X

- **Xeno-transplantation:** Transplantation of organs from one species to another.

Y

- **Yersinia: A** type of bacteria, some of which can cause plague.

Z

- **Zoonosis:** Disease transmissible from animals to humans.

This glossary provides an introduction to some essential medical terms, but medical terminology is vast and complex. It is recommended that you consult specialist sources for more in-depth definitions.

Resources for continuing education.

Continuing education is essential for healthcare professionals. It enables them to keep abreast of medical advances, improve their skills and respond to the changing needs of patients. Here is a list of resources to facilitate continuing education in the medical field:

1. Academic institutions :
   - **Universities and medical schools:** These often offer continuing education programmes for healthcare professionals.
   - **Clinical training centres:** These establishments are specially designed to provide practical training in cutting-edge medical techniques.
2. Professional organisations :
   - **Professional bodies:** They regularly organise seminars, workshops and conferences.
   - **Medical associations:** For example, the World Medical Association and the American Medical Association offer resources and training programmes.
3. Online platforms :
   - **MOOCs:** Platforms such as Coursera, edX and Udemy offer courses on a variety of medical subjects.
   - **Webinars:** Many organisations offer live or recorded webinars for training purposes.
4. Professional publications :
   - **Medical journals:** Publications such as the "New England Journal of Medicine" or "The Lancet" present the latest research.
   - **Professional newsletters:** These resources provide regular updates on trends and developments in the field.
5. Workshops and conferences :
   - **Local seminars:** These events offer the opportunity to learn in an interactive way.

- **National and international conferences:** These provide an opportunity to hear from world experts and network with other professionals.

6. Institutional resources :
   - **Research centres:** These can offer training programmes on new research techniques.
   - **Hospitals and clinics:** These establishments may have in-house programmes to train their staff.
7. Specialised training :
   - **Certification courses:** For specialist skills, for example in medical imaging or robotic surgery.
   - **Practical workshops:** Sessions where professionals can practise new skills under the supervision of experts.
8. Government resources :
   - **National health agencies:** such as the FDA in the United States or the ANSM in France, which can offer resources and training on regulations and guidelines.
9. Books and manuals :
   - **Academic publications:** Many publishers produce books on medical advances, clinical guidelines and best practice.
10. Professional social networks :
    - **Forums and groups:** On platforms such as LinkedIn or ResearchGate, where professionals can exchange information, ask questions and share resources.

Continuing education is a long-term investment for all healthcare professionals. Not only does it guarantee better quality care for patients, it also reinforces the professional's confidence and expertise in his or her field.

Further reading.

A solid bibliography is essential if you want to learn more about endocrinology. Here is a list of recommended books and journals for those wishing to delve deeper into this field:

Books :

"Williams Textbook of Endocrinology" by Shlomo Melmed, Ronald Koenig, et al.

An essential reference covering the fundamental and clinical aspects of endocrinology.

"Endocrinology: Adult and Pediatric" by J. Larry Jameson and Leslie J. De Groot.

A comprehensive book on endocrinology for adult and paediatric   patients.

"Greenspan's Basic & Clinical Endocrinology" by David G. Gardner and Dolores Shoback.

A concise but thorough introduction to clinical endocrinology.

"Clinical Endocrinology and Diabetes: An Illustrated Colour Text" by Miles Levy, Andrew Lansdown, and Robert D. Murray.

A visually engaging book that provides an introduction to clinical endocrinology and diabetes.

"The Thyroid and Its Diseases: A Comprehensive Guide for the Clinician" by Markus Luster, Leonidas H. Duntas, and Leonard Wartofsky.

A book focusing on the thyroid, one of the most essential glands in the endocrine system.

Magazines :

"The Journal of Clinical Endocrinology & Metabolism (JCEM)".

A leading journal that publishes original research on clinical endocrinology.

"Endocrine Reviews
    Provides in-depth reviews of current research in endocrinology.
"European Journal of Endocrinology
    Covers a wide range of subjects related to clinical and fundamental endocrinology.
"Hormone Research in Paediatrics
    Focusing on paediatric endocrinology, this journal is a valuable resource for professionals working with children.
"Thyroid
    A journal dedicated to thyroid research, from fundamental aspects to clinical applications.
Online resources :
    Endocrine Society (www.endocrine.org)
        Offers a variety of resources, including clinical guidelines, webinars and online courses.
    American Association of Clinical Endocrinologists (www.aace.com)
        Provides guidelines, training and information on upcoming conferences.

When looking for resources, it's always a good idea to check the publication date to make sure the information is up-to-date, especially in a constantly evolving field like endocrinology.

The French-speaking world is also full of solid references on endocrinology. Here is a list of recommended books and journals for those wishing to deepen their knowledge in this field:

Books :

    "Endocrinology, diabetology and nutrition" by Jacques Young and Marc Lombès.

- This book provides an overview of the various endocrine disorders, from their molecular basis to their clinical aspects.

"Endocrinology in gynaecology and obstetrics" by Philippe Bouchard and Roland Paillet.

- This book explores the links between endocrinology and gynaecology, including hormonal disorders during pregnancy.

"Clinical Diabetology" by Claude Colette and Alain Golay.

- A comprehensive guide to diabetes, its management and complications.

"Endocrine glands and their mysteries" by Jean-François Pradat.

- A more general approach aimed at non-professionals who want to understand the role of the endocrine glands.

Magazines :

- "Annals of Endocrinology
  - A scientific journal dedicated to endocrinology, covering basic and clinical research.
- "Medicine of Metabolic Diseases
  - Focusing on metabolic diseases, including those linked to hormonal imbalances.
- "Diabetes & Metabolism
  - As its name suggests, this journal focuses on diabetes and other metabolic disorders.

Online resources :

- French Society of Endocrinology (SFE) (www.sfendocrino.org)
  - Provides a range of resources for professionals, including recommendations, training and news on endocrinology in France.
- Association Francophone du Diabète (AFD) (www.afd.asso.fr)
  - A valuable source of information on diabetes in the French-speaking world.

French Federation of Diabetics (www.federationdesdiabetiques.org)

Provides information, resources and news about diabetes.